Issues in Pacific/Asian American

HEALTH AND MENTAL HEALTH

Report of a P/AAMHRC Task Force

P/AAMHRC OCCASIONAL PAPER SERIES
No. 8

Other publications in the series:

Issues in Pacific/Asian American

HEALTH AND MENTAL HEALTH

Report of a P/AAMHRC Task Force

Edited by

Alice K. Murata
Judith Farquhar

Occasional Paper No. 8

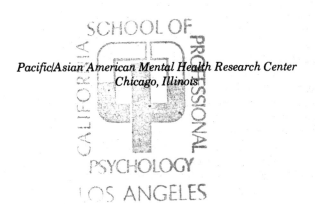

Pacific/Asian American Mental Health Research Center
Chicago, Illinois

International Standard Book Number 0-934584-10-9.
Library of Congress Catalog Number 82-3507.

Prepared under DHEW Grants 5 R01 MH25589 and 1 R01 MH 32820,
and DHHS Grant 7 R01 MH36408.

Library of Congress Cataloging in Publication Data
Main entry under title:

Issues in Pacific/Asian American health and mental health.

    (Occasional paper ; no. 8)
    Bibliography: p
    Contents: Mortality among foreign- and native-born Chinese in
the United States / Haitung King -- Mental health needs of Asian
Americans and Pacific islanders / Joe Yamamoto -- Mental health
delivery system to Asian Americans / Soon-Hyung Chung -- [etc.]
    1. Asian Americans--Medical care. 2. Oceanian Americans--
Medical care. 3. Asian Americans--Mental health services.
4. Oceanian Americans--Mental health services. 5. Health
behavior--United States.
    I. Murata, Alice K. II. Farquhar, Judith.
    III. Pacific/Asian American Mental Health Research Center. IV.
Series: Occasional paper (Pacific/Asian American Mental Health
Research Center) ; no. 8.
RA448.5.A83I77   362.1'08995073   82-3507
ISBN 0-934584-10-9   AACR2

CONTENTS

A Note on the P/AAMHRC
Health and Mental Health Task Force

The Pacific/Asian American Mental Health Research Center (P/AAMHRC) has been funded since 1974 by a grant awarded through the National Institute of Mental Health's Center for Minority Group Mental Health Programs. The purposes of P/AAMHRC are to identify, initiate, conduct, and administer research in areas affecting the well-being and mental health of Pacific/Asian Americans. The organization has a national community advisory committee, and is affiliated with the University of Illinois at Chicago.

Initially, research priorities of the Center were established with reference to community needs and by decision of its community-based board. The first major priority areas to be identified were aging, economic conditions, immigration, and negative stereotypes, and task forces of experts from the Pacific/Asian American communities were convened to develop position papers on each subject. In 1977-1978, a fifth priority area was added, health and mental health, and a task force was formed to undertake a preliminary review of subjects under this heading. What follow are the reports and position papers prepared by members of this body in 1978, with an introduction that summarizes additional insights gained from discussion.

CONTRIBUTORS

Soon-Hyung Chung, a psychiatrist with the State of Hawaii Adult Judiciary System, Courts and Corrections Branch. (Korean).

Lydia Dantes, a nurse on the teaching staff of the University of Illinois School of Nursing. (Pilipino).

Anthony Ishisaka, social worker, program consultant to the Asian Counselling and Referral Service in Seattle. (Japanese).

Haitung King, epidemiologist, National Cancer Institute, Bethesda, Maryland. (Chinese).

Jane F. Lee, a physician in private practice and on the Board of Medical Quality Assurance, Division of Licensing, State of California. (Chinese).

Joe Okimoto, task force chairman, a psychiatrist at the Veterans Administration Hospital and at the University of Washington, Seattle. (Japanese).

Hernan M. Reyes, Chief of Surgery, Cook County (Illinois) Childrens' Hospital. (Pilipino).

Joe Yamamoto, a psychiatrist, chief of UCLA Adult Ambulatory Care Services, director of the Los Angeles Asian/Pacific Counselling Clinic. (Japanese).

Introduction

Recently, popular pressure for health care reform in America from many quarters has increased dramatically. A growing consumer activism, especially among women, handicapped, and families of chronically ill and dying patients, has pointed out the extent to which public needs are not being adequately met by the professional health and mental health system. Discriminated against and underserved by most of our nation's large institutions, America's minorities are now joining in this health care reform movement, voicing their concern that access to decent medical care should not be blocked by language barriers and official ethnocentrism.

Asian Americans are heterogeneous in the extreme, but they have much in common with other Americans who are not satisfied with our current health care system. In seeking the common ground of the Asian and Pacific Islander minorities in America, many issues are raised that extend beyond the needs of these special interest groups. An examination of these needs can clarify the ways in which our medical system has failed, and the areas in which reform might improve real services to those who need them.

Legislation now pending in Congress for some form of unified national health insurance plan is sure to have a fundamental impact on the organization of our medical system in the future; it will also affect the directions of innovation and reform. It is therefore especially urgent that underserved minorities make their health and mental health needs known now. In the case of Pacific/Asian Americans, it is necessary not only to articulate for policy consideration the most obvious needs of our diverse communities; it is also necessary to stimulate more research into the health and mental health conditions among these populations.

The P/AAMHRC health and mental health task force--whose papers are collected herein--met with two purposes: 1) to develop a Pacific/Asian position with relation to current policy issues, and 2) to set priorities and offer guidelines for much-needed research on Asians and Pacific Islanders living in the United States.

The papers collected in this volume reflect the relative lack of systematic knowledge about the health of these ethnic minority groups. At best, illness mortality data are available only for Japanese, Chinese, and Filipino Americans, so that it is difficult to make even rough estimates of the health status of such rapidly growing groups as new immigrants from Korea, Indochina, and South Asia. Where data is less readily available for all groups--e.g., with respect to non-fatal illness or behavioral disorders, the isolation of

1

many Asian American communities from the mainstream of American society has impeded survey research. Important methodological questions concerning social science research on ethnic minorities have been raised by this situation. They must be resolved as the gaps in our knowledge of Asian Americans are bridged.

The task force thus faced a quite open-ended "task." Its members had all had extensive first-hand experience with various Asian American communities, and they perceived many specific needs and problems. But they also realized that systematic research on the health and mental health of these groups had seldom gone beyond either limited studies oriented toward social service needs assessment, or survey research with small samples and inadequate instruments. They sought in their discussions to elucidate areas in which more reliable and detailed information is needed, as well as to explore the basis on which an informed position can be taken now regarding public policy as it affects Pacific/Asian Americans.

HEALTH

As is shown by the epidemiological summary of mortality among Chinese in the United States provided by task force member Haitung King, there is no reason to assume that Asian Americans are an especially healthy segment of our population. Dr. King's paper makes it very clear that the health profile of Chinese Americans is different not only from that of the general U.S. population, but that there are significant differences in some conditions between the generations of Chinese immigrant families. Unfortunately, studies in which such large bodies of data could be drawn upon and in which such factors as generational differences could be isolated are not possible with most other Pacific/Asian groups, due to the inadequacy of long-term mortality data that record ethnic differences. But just such studies as these can teach us something about the health effects of immigration, the role of culture-specific life-styles (e.g., nutritional habits) in illness patterns, and the existence of biogenetic factors in certain diseases that are still little understood.

It is also important to note that, if our health care system is in the process of developing an emphasis on prevention rather than on disease intervention, population biology and epidemiology of the sort that Dr. King has done will form an essential research base for such a service delivery policy. For example, in the case of a chronic fatal disease such as cancer of the nasopharynx (found in high incidence in Chinese populations around the world), ethnically focused public health screening programs for early detection and treatment might be found to be in order. First, however, much more will have to be understood about clusters of environmental influences and genetic factors that increase the probability of any individual developing specific diseases. Careful studies of ethnic enclaves in comparison with the wider U.S. population and with their countries of origin could be a major contribution to this research effort.

Some of the obvious and knotty questions that are raised by a new emphasis on life-style factors and on disease prevention are addressed in the appendix to this report, "Holistic Health: A Public Policy." Many of these questions will require answers based more on ethical and political developments than on research findings, but information regarding the health characteristics of our various ethnic minorities must form an essential precondition to the gradual achievement of a truly preventive medical service delivery system.

This point cannot be emphasized too strongly in view of the dramatic rise in the proparation of total mortality that is attributable to chronic illnesses such as cancer and cerebrovascular and coronary disorders. Dr. King's paper shows that there is a gradual tendency for immigrant groups to take on this illness pattern that is characteristic of American society. Increasingly, prevention is the only hope for "cure" of our major medical problems, and all Americans will be affected by consequent reorientation of our medical care system.

Some of the apparently group-specific high incidence health problems cited by King are, in theory at least, more preventable and understandable than nasopharyngeal cancer. Causes of death such as suicide and homicide are higher among Chinese Americans than among their Asian counterparts; we must assume that such health problems are at least potentially preventable, and close investigation of the social setting in which deaths from these causes occur is urgently indicated. Preliminary evidence suggests that suicide among aged Chinese is often linked with chronic illness and unwillingness to seek medical care. We suspect that this is only one symptom of a deep-seated collection of social and personal problems faced by Asian aged people in the U.S., which urgently require both research and social service attention. Health problems cannot really be separated from social conditions. This principle holds especially true not only for Pacific/Asian Americans, but also for all disadvantaged groups in the U.S.

MENTAL HEALTH

The mental health conditions and needs of Pacific/Asian Americans were examined by Drs. Joe Yamamoto and Soon-Hyung Chung, both of them clinicians with years of experience in developing appropriate therapies for Asian Americans. For both of them, the stigma attached to mental illness and to the seeking of mental health services was a major concern. Some reasons cited for this apparently abnormal level of shame related to the need for mental health services included: 1) differences between explanatory models used in the Far East and in the U.S., such that mental illness is perceived to be a characterological defect by Americans while it is more often seen as a transitory illness by Asians; 2) concern about immigration status and official racism, in that behavioral deviance among Asian Americans could jeopardize their ability to stay in this country or to succeed in American society; and 3) a strong emphasis on family responsibility for ailing members, with shame resulting from unacceptable behavior being attached to the whole family and encouraging a tendency to hide disturbed individuals.

Both Yamamoto and Chung have observed a tendency among their patients to express psychological disorders in terms of somatic illness; there are various ways of understanding and learning from this phenomenon, and recent literature in medical anthropology and sociology has begun to propose useful approaches. It is an area that can be very productively studied; it is also, however, a characteristic of Asian American health behavior that should be understood by medical and mental health service providers. A tendency to present somatic complaints instead of psychological ones demands not only sensitivity to the phenomenon but also innovative clinical responses.

Certain subgroups among Pacific/Asian Americans are especially subject to stress as a result of their social situation; preliminary evidence indicates that these same groups are more likely to develop symptoms requiring mental health treatment. Recent immigrants and the elderly constitute the most numerous populations in this category. New immigrants to the U.S. are afflicted with much more subtle pressures than the obvious difficulties presented by language barriers, money problems, and employment discrimination. They are also especially affected by racism and by the effects of culturally sanctioned behavior patterns (such as nonaggressiveness) that prove to be maladaptive in the American setting. Such factors as these combined with the frequent isolation of immigrant individuals and families from others sharing their cultural background can (and apparently far too often do) result in considerable distress.

It is worth noting that the differential psychological effects of the "ghettoization" of Chinese and Japanese migrants to the U.S. in the past has been little studied in comparison with the geographic scattering that is a feature of some more recent arrivals from Asia and the Pacific. There is, however, a clear tendency among Southeast Asian refugees, who were systematically scattered throughout the U.S. on first arrival, to migrate to areas on the West Coast, where noticeable ethnic communities are developing. This phenomenon points to the role of community support groups in easing the tensions of immigration, and should be carefully monitored with an eye to its effect on rates of behavioral disorder in the ethnic groups involved. (This is a component of the ongoing research work of P/AAMHRC).

The problems of Asian and Pacific American elderly people are less clearly related to recent arrival in the U.S., although they are perhaps more acute among new immigrants. Cultural attitudes to the family and the individual among Asian groups differ markedly from mainstream American cultural values, and such attitudes appear to be very deep-seated and stable. Research on Japanese American families which have been here long enough to have adult third-generation American members (Sansei) indicates that these differences in Asian and American cultures continue to produce high levels of stress within such families. Elderly members of Asian families seem to be particularly affected by the discontinuity between the way in which they expected to grow old, with dignity and power accorded to them by their relatives by virtue of their seniority, and the way in which aging takes place in America. Furthermore, the plight of many Asians and Pacific Islanders who are separated from or have lost their families (examples are single refugees and men who immigrated to the U.S. to find work) is only worsened by the social conditions attendant upon aging in America.

A family- and community-oriented approach in mental health service delivery has been frequently referred to in the research and social work literature on Asian American ethnic conditions. Problems such as those discussed above would clearly be effectively addressed by sensitive and imaginative application of such techniques as family therapy and by a more effective interface between mental health service personnel and community agencies. We would emphasize, however, that lip service given to the importance of social and cultural factors in services to Pacific/Asian Americans is not enough. Ideally, specialized services provided by experienced and innovative practitioners who share the native language and ethnic background of their clients should be available. Failing this, much more research and training on social and cultural factors in mental illness, along with a much broader emphasis on bilingual services in mental health agencies, would improve our understanding of and our services to our ethnic minorities. Improved outreach and public education programs are also recommended as an approach to addressing the tendency by Asians to underutilize available mental health services due to the high level of stigma attached to mental illness. Dr. Chung's successful experience with a problem-solving television show, and Dr. Yamamoto's heavily utilized Asian American clinic, both indicate that there is much room for improvement along the lines discussed here.

PROFESSIONAL LICENSING

A public policy issue that is closely related to the health and mental health research and service problems cited above is that of manpower training and licensing. While those concerned with service delivery to Pacific/Asian Americans call for practitioners who are culturally and linguistically suited to the clients, there are many Asian and Pacific foreign medical graduates who are unable to obtain licensure to practice in the areas for which they have been trained.

Dr. Lee's thorough study of manpower training and licensing problems (somewhat abridged herein) identifies many areas in which official practice could be rendered more equitable and consistent from state to state. It is clear from her report that licensing is easiest for foreign health professionals in states where the overall number of practitioners is lowest relative to total population--i.e., where physicians are in greatest demand. Such total population considerations, however, completely neglect the needs of special populations within each state. Thus, states like California, Illinois, and New York could be considered to have a shortage of health personnel relative to the high proportions of Asians in their populations, especially with regard to poor residents of inner city ethnic enclaves. It would be in the interest of such states to alter their licensing policies to admit more foreign-trained Asian and Pacific medical personnel into practice, and to provide training programs to enable such professionals to meet the quality standards that are protected by the licensing system.

Even apart from considerations of a social need for medical services, the difficulties and complexities for foreign medical graduates of obtaining post-graduate training and licensure must be dealt with at a national policy level. There is little doubt that these obstacles are in part racist in origin and that they run counter to humane immigration principles. Once foreign medical graduates are enabled to compete on an equal basis with U.S. graduates, their needs for further training where applicable will be more clear. Equal opportunity in professional employment should encourage the development of training and orientation programs that can assure licensing boards and patients of the adequacy of the medical services delivered.

Some form of official recognition of culture-specific alternative therapies such as acupuncture could also vastly increase utilization of health services by underserved Asian groups, and improve compliance with clinical programs. As long as official rejection of the medical systems that are characteristic of some of our most numerous minorities is continued, they are forced to be perceived as alternatives rather than as complementary parts of decent medical care. Acupuncture, herbalism, chiropractic, and the "psychotherapy" of spirit healers have become part of a kind of health underground in America which is much more widespread than most medical policy-makers would like to acknowledge. Some form of official recognition and cooperation (e.g., partial insurance coverage, referrals by physicians for ailments they deem to be "psychosomatic" or untreatable by standard medical procedures, and assessment of dietary and health maintenance practices of patients who are using "folk" therapies) between standard medicine and alternative practice might be in order. Such accommodation to the treatment preferences of ethnic patients could have the effect of relieving physicians of minor ailments that they cannot efficiently treat while producing a much greater possibility that patients will be cooperative and satisfied within the overall medical system.

NATIONAL HEALTH LEGISLATION

Most of the popular attention that has been focused on legislation regarding national health insurance has revolved around the interests of physicians in private practice, insurance companies, and the poor and aged people who require special consideration in any such plan. The interests of America's ethnic communities and recent immigrants are not necessarily the same as any of these, however, and demand special consideration at a time when large-scale health reform is being considered. Dr. Reyes's paper in this collection reviews two contrasting approaches to national health insurance; generally speaking, these reflect the National Health Service model and the Universal Health Insurance model. Both models have advantages and disadvantages for Pacific/Asian Americans, some of which are not immediately obvious.

A National Health Service in which government would, in part at least, go into the "business" of health care delivery, would, we suspect, resist any introduction of alternative modes of healing such as those discussed above. It might, however, have the capability of introducing fundamental changes in the entire health care delivery system that would correct some of the subtle barriers that have prevented many Asians from getting adequate care up to now. Under sufficient popular pressure, for instance, a national health service could allocate considerable resources from elsewhere in government to provide bilingual services wherever they are needed. Such sweeping change is not likely to take place with a federally-based insurance system, which would essentially leave our medical care and public health systems as they now stand. Similarly, a shift in the emphasis of health care to a preventive model would be facilitated by the introduction of a unified medical service in which organizational policy could be consistent at all levels.

An insurance system, on the other hand, if it were sufficiently flexible, could foster medical pluralism and better enable a consumer-oriented system. In such a system, services that are perceived to be needed by America's various communities and interest groups could be freely developed and utilized, subject to a minimum of federal regulation. This somewhat idealized picture probably comes closer to what many Asian and Pacific American leaders would like, but it remains to be seen which form of federally-assisted medical system is most likely to take account of the needs of Pacific/Asian Americans.

The task force felt that any sweeping health care reform legislation should incorporate the following governing principles:

1) Universality of access, to citizens and non-citizens as well as visitors and people in all immigration statuses.

2) Emphasis on prevention, including public education and outreach as well as public health screening for population specific disorders.

3) Comprehensiveness of services, including increased use of "mid-level extenders" (e.g. paramedical personnel) and "alternative" practitioners.

4) Ease of access, with an emphasis on neighborhood family health centers and continuing education for practitioners in social and cultural issues relating to health care delivery.

In general, the health insurance model was favored over the national health service model, with the hope that a very wide range of services would be reimbursable under its provisions. As envisioned here, plurality of available services could be fostered under such a system such that Asian and Pacific American clients could "shop" for services where they feel most certain of being effectively helped. This is a "fee for services" model in the widest sense, since the task force firmly supports the full utilization of health maintenance organizations, family practice clinics, health screening agencies, the utilization of paramedical and social work personnel, and the integration of alternative healers into the health care network. The ultimate goal is to preserve and foster medical pluralism without sacrificing quality care as a service to America's extremely diverse ethnic populations who are at present underserved as a result of poverty, mistrust, and bureaucratic apathy.

In this introduction we have tried to provide a context into which the specific issues raised by each of the papers collected here can be placed. The large questions that are yet to be resolved regarding the health conditions and needs of America's Asian and Pacific minority people are many and complex, and they are only touched on in this volume. We hope, however, that the dialogue on the health and mental health needs of special populations in the U.S. is only beginning, and that Pacific/Asian American voices will increasingly be heard within it.

CHAPTER 1
Mortality Among Foreign- and Native-Born Chinese in the United States

Haitung King, PhD

The first immigrant group to the U.S. from Asia was the Chinese, who started arriving in the U.S. in large numbers around 1850. For this reason, the largest and oldest group of U.S.-born Asian Americans are Chinese; they are the only Asian American population in which epidemiological studies of the long-term health effects of immigration can yield significant results in comparison with the general U.S. population. Dr. King reports below that mortality from various causes among Chinese Americans is approaching that of their white counterparts, with some interesting exceptions. This study is important not only with reference to Chinese Americans, but also because of the overview it provides of the effects of immigration on the health of America's minority populations.

Epidemiological studies of the Chinese populations at home and abroad are relatively few, and most of them are limited in scope and/or method. In the United States, the first known mortality study of the Chinese was initiated by Winslow and Koh in 1924. This was followed 20 years later by a cursory investigation of the health of the Chinese in San Francisco (Geiger, 1945). More recent studies, notably those of Smith (1956) and King and Haenszel (1973), dealt exclusively with malignant neoplasms.

In view of the need for a systematic ascertainment of the overall health status of the Chinese in the United States, this paper examines mortality from selected major diseases and causes of death among foreign- and native-born Chinese, 1959-1962. In earlier decades, the U.S.-born population over age 45 was too small to warrant investigation of nativity differentials in risk of chronic diseases. By 1960, 16 and 11 percent of U.S.-born males and females had reached this age, respectively, thus permitting a review of mortality by nativity. (Table 1).

A conventional practice denotes the first generation of Japanese migrating to the United States as Issei and their U.S.-born descendants as Nisei. To facilitate discussion, the counterpart terms idai and erdai have been coined for the foreign- and U.S.-born

Table 1. Percentage Distribution of Population by Sex and Nativity, U.S. Chinese, 1960

Sex and Age (in years)	Idai	Erdai
Males		
Total number	59,083	76,347
0-4	0.7	18.1
5-14	5.3	30.5
15-24	10.1	11.3
25-34	19.0	13.4
35-44	20.3	10.7
45-54	18.8	6.5
55-64	15.2	5.5
65-74	7.9	2.8
75 and over	2.7	1.2
Females		
Total number	34,205	66,449
0-4	1.3	19.7
5-14	7.8	31.7
15-24	13.2	12.5
25-34	28.3	14.0
35-44	19.6	11.1
45-54	14.6	6.0
55-64	9.4	3.4
65-74	4.4	1.3
75 and over	1.4	0.3

SOURCE: U.S. Bureau of Commerce, 1963, Tables 4, 7 and 8.

Chinese (i in Chinese means one, and er, two; in Japanese ichi and ni; dai, meaning generation, is comparable to the Japanese sei). For more specific contrasts between the second and third generation of Chinese Americans, the term sandai is suggested to parallel the Japanese equivalent, Sansei.

SOURCES OF DATA

Mortality data for the U.S. Chinese are based on special tabulations of deaths, 1959-1962. For comparison with the Chinese in Asia, mortality statistics for comparable years were obtained from the health offices in Taiwan, Hong Kong, and Singapore. The findings on the last three populations will be referred to in the discussion but are not shown in the tables.

The 1960 U.S. Census enumeration was used to estimate the Chinese-American population at risk for 1959-1962. Judging from the percent distribution by sex, age, and nativity, the effect of legal and social restrictions imposed since the 1850s upon the Chinese immigrants (King, unpublished paper) were clearly reflected in the high male-female ratio (1.3:1), and the heavy concentration of idai Chinese at ages 25 and over. The smaller proportion of idai females (33 percent) was related in part to "sojourner" attitudes of early Chinese immigrants. The sojourn was a "job" to be completed within the shortest possible time, with no intention of remaining permanently in the host country. However, the major influence stemmed from the legal prohibition against Chinese laborers bringing in their wives. The current peak of idai females at age 25 to 34 (28 percent) mirrored the influx since 1943 of war brides and of female relatives of Chinese Americans following repeal of the Chinese Exclusion Act of 1882.

The 1960 census data also revealed a high concentration of Chinese in urban areas (96 percent), mainly in San Francisco, New York City, Honolulu, and Los Angeles. Other notable characteristics included a relatively small proportion of "ever-married, spouse absent" among erdai males and a low educational attainment among their idai counterparts. Further, the idai male labor force was concentrated in such industries as wholesale and retail trade and personal services.

It must be pointed out that, in spite of the negative stereotype of the Chinese in the minds of the general public, this population as a whole had in 1969 a high median family income of $6,207, being second only to the Japanese ($6,842) but higher than the whites ($5,893) and other groups (Kitagawa and Hauser, 1973).

METHODS OF STUDY

Standardized mortality ratios (SMRs) were used to measure the mortality level of the Chinese. An SMR is the ratio of the number of deaths observed among the Chinese population to the number of deaths expected, on the basis of the 1959-1961 age-specific death rates of U.S. white males and females, the "standard population." The "standard population" has the value 100 percent. The precision of the SMRs is indicated by the computed 95 percent confidence limits (not shown in tables).

In the interpretation of disease-specific mortality differences, both the summarized SMRs and the overall patterns of age-specific mortality (not shown in paper) are considered. It must be noted that, because of the comparatively small number of observed deaths, the SMRs for U.S. Chinese females are most subject to sampling variation.

MAJOR FINDINGS

GENERAL MORTALITY
    According to Winslow and Koh (Table 2), the crude rate for all combined causes of death among the U.S. Chinese of both sexes in 1921 was more than twice that of the white population. By 1949-1951, mortality differences between U.S. Chinese and whites were greatly reduced. The standardized mortality ratios for Chinese males and females, based on the age-specific death rates of whites, were shown to be 130 and 113, respectively. During the study period of our investigation, 1959-1962, the SMR for Chinese males practically approached the level of their white counterparts, whereas the SMR for Chinese females was deficient by 17 percent (Table 3). The more favorable ratio for 1959-1962 over 1949-1951 was mainly attributable to the reduced mortality from causes with large numbers of deaths such as circulatory diseases.

Table 2. Crude Death Rates Per 100,000 by Selected Major Causes, U.S. Chinese in the Registration States, 1921

Cause of Death	Rate	Ratio[a] White=100
All causes	2,447.2	218
Tuberculosis	526.3	617
Circulatory system	332.8	183
External cause	332.8	382
Respiratory system	238.8	232
Genitourinary system	202.6	210
Nervous system	173.6	142
Digestive system	164.6	149
Early infancy	45.2	68
Congenital malformation	14.5	90
Skin and cellular tissue	10.9	287
Puerperal state	3.6	23

SOURCE: Winslow and Koh, 1924.

[a] Computed by this author.

The idai males showed a much higher mortality than their erdai counterparts for all causes combined and for most specific diseases (Tables 4 and 5). However, some of the SMRs exhibited wide differences of confidence limits. A similar, although smaller disparity appeared in the female data, but the number of observations was usually small. The higher idai SMRs were attributed to their higher rates at older ages. For example, the idai age-sex-specific mortality for all combined causes was ten times higher than those for erdai among males age 65 to 74 and among females 75 years and over.

Table 3. SMRs for Selected Broad Disease Groups, U.S. Chinese, 1949-1952 and 1959-1962 (U.S. White Males and Females, 1950-1951 and 1959-1961 Equal 100)

	Male		Female	
Cause of Death	1949-1952	1959-1962	1949-1952	1959-1962
All causes	130	100	113	83
Infective and parasitic	425	276	142	119
Malignant neoplasms	131	121	101	94
Nervous system and sense organs	119	100	118	82
Circulatory system	103	80	92	74
Respiratory system	165	127	148	75
Digestive system	195	158	69	58
Certain diseases of early infancy	119	75	122	60
Accidents, poisonings, and violence	98	78	136	93

SOURCE: Adapted from King, 1975; Smith, 1956.

Table 4. SMRs for Selected Causes of Death, U.S. Chinese, 1959-1962 (U.S. White Males and Females, 1959-1961 Equal 100)

Cause of Death	Male Idai	Male Erdai	Female Idai	Female Erdai
All causes	115	78	96	71
Tuberculosis	444	198	180	n.c.
Cancer	137	97	106	77
Diabetes	232	145	138	98
Stroke	114	85	97	68
Heart, coronary	69	65	64	55
Hypertension, heart	224	190	184	96
Hypertension, other	147	83	n.c.	231
Pneumonia	222	96	89	68
Ulcer, stomach	391	106	276	n.c.
Ulcer, duodenum	170	83	n.c.	n.c.
Cirrhosis of liver	248	62	n.c.	n.c.
Nephritis, nephrosis	223	165	189	173
Accidents, motor	73	32	72	51
Accidents, other	75	46	78	50
Suicide	174	76	407	118
Homicide	235	129	53	n.c.

SOURCE: Adapted from King, 1975

n.c. Fewer than 5 deaths; SMR not computed.

Table 5. SMRs for Selected Cancer Sites, U.S. Chinese,
1959-1962 (U.S. White Males and Females, 1959-1961 Equal
100)

Site of Cancer	Male Idai	Male Erdai	Female Idai	Female Erdai
All sites	137	97	106	77
Nasopharynx	3,435	2,500	2,940	n.c.
Esophagus	294	191	n.c.	n.c.
Stomach	137	108	187	116
Intestines	130	71	75	65
Rectum	131	87	109	n.c.
Liver, primary	1,273	870	n.c.	n.c.
Pancreas	102	94	78	n.c.
Trachea, lung and bronchus	135	85	226	311
Breast	n.a.	n.a.	61	34
Cervix uteri	n.a.	n.a.	67	83
Other uterus	n.a.	n.a.	127	n.c.
Ovary	n.a.	n.a.	70	100
Prostate	29	35	n.a.	n.a.
Bladder and other urinary organs	67	62	n.c.	n.c.
Skin	66	n.c.	n.c.	n.c.
Brain and nervous system	57	58	n.c.	n.c.
Lymphosarcoma, etc.	94	82	102	120
Leukemia and aleukemia	50	97	187	83

SOURCE: Adapted from King and Haenszel, 1973.

n.a. Not applicable.

n.c. Fewer than 5 deaths; SMR not computed.

CARDIOVASCULAR-RENAL DISEASES

Coronary heart disease and hypertension: Compared to their Asian counterparts, idai and erdai of both sexes showed an elevated mortality for coronary heart disease. The upward displacement was in accord with the experience of the Japanese migrants to the United States (Haenszel and Kurihara, 1968). The SMRs for the four U.S. Chinese nativity-sex groups were more than twice those for the Asian Chinese. Such an elevation brought the mortality level for the U.S. Chinese up to about two-thirds as high as that for the host population. In view of the smaller range of differences for this disease between U.S. Chinese and whites aged 65 and over, a further rise among the Chinese might be predicted.

As with the migrants from Japan, there was generally a rise in mortality among the U.S. Chinese for hypertensive heart disease and other hypertensive diseases combined. However, the Chinese pattern differed from that of the U.S. Chinese in that the SMRs greatly exceeded those for the host country.

Vascular lesions: The apparent reduction in mortality from strokes shown for the U.S. Chinese was in keeping with the mortality experience of the Japanese migrants to the United States (Haenszel and Kurihara, 1968). The age-specific patterns of the nativity sex-groups were consistent with the impression conveyed by the summary SMRs.

Nephritis and Nephrosis: Mortality from nephritis and nephrosis remained high among the U.S. Chinese, in spite of a downward transition. The age-specific patterns of the U.S. Chinese showed a sharp rise in mortality at about age 55 and over, and the curves became steeper with age thereafter.

MALIGNANT NEOPLASMS

The cancer mortality experience of the U.S. Chinese was relatively stable from 1949-1952 to 1959-1962, following the prevailing trend for U.S. whites during those years (Table 3).

The known high liability of the Chinese to nasopharyngeal cancer was amplified by our findings, the SMRs for idai Chinese being 30 times higher than for white males and females. Other notable characteristics of the Chinese from the vantage point of internal U.S. comparisons were the low risk for prostate and high risk for liver and esophagus among males, and the low risk for breast and high risk for lung among females.

For all combined cancer sites, a significantly higher SMR was shown for idai than erdai males. A similar but less marked disparity was exhibited for females. Higher idai male SMRs were noted for most specific cancer sites, but the wide confidence limits made it difficult to identify those with firmly established differentials, especially for the females. Colon and lung were the two sites for which higher risks among idai males were most strongly suggested. Age-specific data indicated that higher idai death rates at older ages contributed to their higher SMRs.

SUICIDE, HOMICIDE, AND ACCIDENT

Suicide: For suicide, the SMRs for idai of both sexes exceeded those for Chinese in Hong Kong and Singapore, whereas the SMRs for erdai were low to approximately the level of U.S. whites. The age-specific rates pointed in the same direction, indicating a particularly steep rise for idai aged 55 years and over. No such an early elevation was observed among erdai, or most Chinese elders, who usually command high status and respect in the family and community. In contrast, the life of aged idai, particularly males in Chinatowns, are likely to be characterized by isolation, loneliness, destitution, and ill health, in addition to loss of status. The findings of a San Francisco study in 1960-1968 (Bourne, 1973) clearly conveyed such an impression. For example, of the 61 Chinese males who committed suicide, 21 were unemployed, another 21 were cooks or retired persons, 5 were skilled laborers, and 7 were laundry and restaurant workers. Further, physical illness was reported to be a predominant cause of suicide in aged Chinese males.

It is interesting to note that, unlike Western and other non-Western countries for which data are available (Segi et al., 1966), a noticeably high mortality from suicide was exhibited in both U.S. and Asian Chinese females, reflecting perhaps their major problems of interpersonal conflict (46 percent for Hong Kong Chinese females committing suicide; Yap, 1958).

It is also noted that "never-married" Chinese males had a higher suicide SMR than their "ever-married" counterparts (152 vs. 116). However, in assessing the mortality differential between these two groups, one must take into account the likely spurious effect arising from marital classifications. Specifically, a large proportion of "ever-married" Chinese males (especially idai in older age groups) were classified as "married, spouse absent", meaning that their wives have remained in the homeland (Table 6). Presumably, these "de facto singles" would have been subjected to the same health risks which afflict "singles de jure." Therefore, inclusion of this "functionally single" group might have had an inflating effect on the mortality of the entire group of "ever married" Chinese males.

Homicide: For homicide among males, a higher SMR was shown for the U.S. Chinese, particularly idai, than for the Asian Chinese. Further, the age-specific curves were noted to be rather irregular and abrupt up into senescence, in contrast to the more smoothly declining slope at early age for the U.S. whites.

Accidents: There was in general a noticeable rise in motor vehicle accidents among the U.S. Chinese, in comparison with the Chinese in Asia. The reverse held true for "other accidents" (except

Table 6.   Percent of Spouse Absent, Married U.S. Chinese
Males 20 years Old and Over, by Nativity and Age, 1960

Age (in years)	Idai	Erdai
All ages	22.7	9.9
20-24	18.0	8.2
25-34	15.2	4.7
35-44	13.2	5.2
45-64	27.6	14.3
65 and over	36.4	23.0

SOURCE: U.S. Department of Commerce, 1963, Tables 22, 30.

Singapore). Also noted was a conspicuous elevation in age-specific rates for "other accidents" among idai males aged 65 years and over. Perhaps some of these cases might have been accidents with undetected suicide motivations.

INFECTIVE, RESPIRATORY, ALIMENTARY,
AND DIABETIC DISEASES
     Infective diseases: The reduction in mortality from tuberculosis among the U.S. Chinese has been impressive. For example, the idai SMRs were depressed as low as one-tenth to one-fifth of that for Hong Kong, even though the male age-specific rates continued to rise to the highest age-bracket. Among erdai males, a considerable reduction occurred at age 55-64 and particularly at age 75 and over. Such a downward transition was understandable considering the differing socioeconomic levels in the host country and home base.
     Respiratory diseases: As with tuberculosis, pneumonia displayed a substantially reduced SMR for the U.S. Chinese, especially for the females.
     Alimentary diseases: Apparently there was a downward transition among the U.S. Chinese in deaths from such alimentary diseases as ulcers of stomach and duodenum and liver cirrhosis. The age-specific curves of cirrhosis of the liver for erdai followed those for the host country rather closely.
     Diabetes: As with few other causes of death, diabetes was another disease exhibiting upward displacement among the U.S. Chinese. The SMRs for all nativity-sex groups, except erdai females, exceeded those for both home and host populations. This impressions was clearly strengthened by the age-specific curves.

DISCUSSION

BASIS OF INTERPRETATION:
A CONCEPTUAL FRAME OF REFERENCE
For a meaningful interpretation of some of the findings presented in this paper and for exploration of suggestive epidemiologic
clues, a conceptual frame of reference is proposed and illustrated in
Figure 1. A full exposition of the scheme is beyond the scope of this
paper; but the underlying rationale may be briefly stated. Basically,
our position is that in comprehensive epidemiologic investigation of
diseases, attention should be directed to three component factors:
biogenetic predisposition, ecological influence, and sociocultural
intervention. Some of the specific variables in each component
group are identified in the scheme. The main emphasis is on the
interaction of these component factors and specific variables.

IMPLICATIONS OF FINDINGS
Of the three types of component factors suggested above,
biogenetic predisposition seems to be the most complex and least
known. In the general absence of convincing biogenetic evidence,
our discussion will be directed to sociocultural intervention and
ecological influence. Such an approach seems to be justified in view
of the noticeable mortality differentials observed between idai and
erdai. Even in the case of nasopharyngeal cancer, for which biogenetic predisposition has generally been implicated because of its

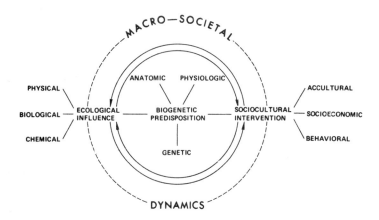

Figure 1. An Epidemiologic Conceptual Scheme for the Study of
Diseases

invariably high prevalence among the Chinese, there were indica-
tions of some reduction in risk from 1949-1952 and 1959-1962. The
lower risk for erdai described in our study, along with the California
findings (Buell, 1965; Zippin, 1962), particularly those pertaining to
sandai (Buell, 1974a), all point to the possible role of nonbiogenetic
factors which remain to be identified.

The trends of female breast cancer further illustrate this
point. Unlike the situation for other migrants to the United States,
there was an absence of risk in female breast cancer mortality
among erdai or Nisei as of 1959-1962 (King and Haenszel, 1973;
Haenszel and Kurihara, 1968). One is naturally tempted to suggest a
role for genetic factors. However, a recent California study (Buell,
1974b) revealed that an increase in incidence did eventually occur
among Nisei during the years 1969-1971. The rise trailed about 20
years behind that for Polish women, most of whom came to the
United States during the same period as the Japanese; both groups of
women migrated from rural areas. It remains to be seen whether a
similar transformation has occurred among the Chinese when the
results are available for 1970.

The implications of the interaction of acculturation with other
component and specific factors, as reflected in the above examples,
may be amplified to characterize the overall absence of clear-cut
nativity differentials in mortality among the U.S. Chinese. Such a
phenomenon may not be related to over-reporting among idai of U.S.
birthplaces in the population census, to differences in composition
between early and recent migrant groups, or to the upward social
and occupational mobility of erdai. Perhaps changes in mortality
risks are not fully expressed among the Chinese until relatively
advanced ages. Data must be accumulated over longer time periods
to establish more firmly cause-specific differentials for this population. The long period required not only signifies that acculturation
in general is a slow process, but also that the Chinese are especially
persistent in adhering to the old ways of living.

Of the various Chinese ways of living, perhaps there has been
more speculation on dietary habits than on any other factors in
relation to coronary heart disease. This is because the low prevalence of this condition among the Chinese is generally held to be
related to their depressed serum cholesterol content. The low
cholesterol level among the Chinese is, in turn, said to be attributable to the Chinese diet, which is low in animal fats. Based on such
reasoning, one would suspect that the higher mortality from
coronary heart diseases among the U.S. Chinese than among their
Asian counterparts would be partly attributable to dietary changes.
Although no significant difference in mortality is yet exhibited
between idai and erdai, a further rise among the latter can be
expected as the degree of acculturation heightens.

Lest it be misunderstood, our emphasis on dietary changes does not preclude the possible influence of all other factors associated with acculturation, including the use of automobiles and disengagement from physical activity. Our observations may be sharpened by examining the rise of coronary heart disease among the U.S. Chinese, as compared to the low level for their Asian counterparts. Such an observation parallels that for colonic cancer but contradicts that for cancer of the stomach. A similar transitional experience was observed by Haenszel and Kurihara (1968) among the U.S. Japanese. This is also in keeping with other international comparisons.

Admittedly, the implications of the above configurations are rather obscure, but they do point to a new dimension of dietary effects on both coronary heart disease and large bowel cancer. This is well demonstrated by a recent study of large bowel cancer in Hawaiian Japanese (Haenszel et al., 1973). The authors argue that the association of excess risk in large bowel cancer with the consumption of beef (as compared with chicken, pork, and fish) among well-acculturated U.S. Japanese suggests the high content of saturated fats in this food. The reason is that such long-chain fatty acids pass to the small intestine. This mechanism is in contrast to the short-chain butyric acid in dairy products which is being absorbed through the gastric mucosae. For example, Seventh Day Adventists, who consume large amounts of dairy products but no beef or other meats, have a low intestinal cancer risk.

SUGGESTED APPROACHES TO RESEARCH

In terms of epidemiologic research, perhaps what is needed most are systematic epidemiologic field studies of various Chinese populations, with particular emphasis on subgroup sociocultural differences. The conceptual scheme suggested above would be useful. Indeed, the Chinese represent a distinctive resource for socioepidemiologic studies. They have migrated to many countries throughout the world, and the diversity in new ecologic background and sociocultural setting may yield clues on the interplay of such forces and biogenetic predisposition in diseases and disorders. The findings of such studies would have much to contribute to intercultural epidemiology in general and to nativity differentials among the Chinese in particular.

We shall not attempt to discuss in this paper the details of such field studies, except to point out that the scope of investigations can be extensive and the specific topics to be covered intricate. For example, it would be advisable to conduct comparative studies of acculturation status and illness patterns between idai and erdai (or sandai). The Holmes-Rahe (1967) quantitative instrument may be used to assess life change in relation to illness experience, as

Bruhn et al. (1972) did in their study of U.S. Italians in a Pennsylvania community. As another example, we turn to epidemiologic studies of accidents in Chinese children. Following Kurokawa (1969), one may hypothesize that acculturated Chinese children have more accidents than the non-acculturated due to the exposure factor, and that those who suffer from acculturation conflict have accidents due to coping factors. Speculations of this sort can contribute much in sharpening our epidemiologic observations.

In view of the wide dispersal of the Chinese in the United States, field work may be initiated in such areas as San Francisco, Honolulu, New York City, Los Angeles, and Chicago where this population in concentrated in sufficient numbers. The first two areas are particularly suitable for pursuing case-control and/or cohort studies of specific diseases such as cancer because they are already covered by comprehensive, population-based tumor registries. The findings for cancer of the nasopharynx warrant special efforts to define the U.S. Chinese population more carefully with respect to place of origin and genetically determined traits. Chinese family and association records might be investigated with this point in mind and a more systematic search for genetic markers that may discriminate between population groups that have come from different localities within China should be considered. Information in genetic markers could have useful applications in the conduct of case-control studies.

REFERENCES

Bourne, P. G.
    1973   "Suicide Among Chinese in San Francisco." American Journal of Public Health 83:744-750.

Bruhn, J. G. et al.
    1972   "Social Readjustment and Illness Patterns; Comparisons Between First, Second and Third Generation Italian-Americans Living in the Same Community." Journal of Psychosomatic Research 16:387-394.

Buell, P.
    1965   "Nasopharynx Cancer in Chinese of California." British Journal of Cancer 19:459-470.
    1974a   "The Effect of Migration on the Risk of Nasopharyngeal Cancer among Chinese." Cancer Research 34:1189-1191.
    1974b   "Changing Incidence of Breast Cancer in Japanese-American Women." Journal of the National Cancer Institute 51:1479-1483.

Geiger, J. C. et al.
1945   "The Health of the Chinese in an American City." San Francisco Health Department. Mimeographed.

Haenszel, W. and M. Kurihara
1968   "Studies of Japanese Migrants. 1. Mortality from Cancer and Other Diseases among Japanese in the United States." Journal of the National Cancer Institute 40:43-68.

Haenszel, W., J. W. Berg, M. Segi, M. Kurihara and F. B. Locke
1973   "Large Bowel Cancer in Hawaiian Japanese." Journal of the National Cancer Institute 51:1765-1779.

Holmes, T. H. and R. H. Rahe
1967   "The Social Readjustment Rating Scale." Journal of Psychosomatic Research 11:213-218.

King, H.
n.d.   "A Century of Chinese Immigration to the United States, 1850-1950." Unpublished paper.

1975   "Selected Epidemiologic Aspects of Major Diseases and Causes of Death among Chinese in the United States and Asia." Pp. 487-550 in A. Kleinman et al. (eds.): Medicine in Chinese Cultures: Comparative Studies of Health Care in Chinese and Other Societies. DHEW Publication No. (NIH) 75-653. Bethesda, Maryland: National Institutes of Health, John E. Fogarty International Center.

King, H. and W. Haenszel
1973   "Cancer Mortality Among Foreign- and Native-born Chinese in the United States." Journal of Chronic Diseases 26:623-646.

Kitagawa, E. M. and P. M. Hauser
1973   Differential Mortality in the United States: A Study of Socioeconomic Epidemiology. Cambridge: Harvard University Press.

Kurokawa, M.
1969   "Acculturation and Childhood Accidents Among Chinese and Japanese Americans." Genetic Psychology Monograph 79:89-159.

Segi, M. et al.
1966   Mortality for Selected Causes in 30 Countries (1950-1961). Sendai, Japan: Tohoku University School of Medicine.

Smith, L.
1956   "Recorded and Expected Mortality Among the Chinese in Hawaii and the United States with Special Reference to Cancer." Journal of the National Cancer Institute 17: 667-676.

U.S. Department of Commerce, Bureau of the Census
1963   "Nonwhite Population by Race, U.S. Census of Population, 1960." Final Report PC(2)-1C. Washington, D.C.: U.S. Government Printing Office.

Winslow, C. E. A. and K. W. Koh
1924   "The Mortality of the Chinese in the United States, Hawaii and the Philippines." Journal of Hygiene 4:330-355.

Yap, P. M.
1958   Suicide in Hong Kong. Hong Kong: Hong Kong University Press.

Zippin, C. et al.
1962   "Studies of Heredity and Environment in Cancer of the Nasopharynx." Journal of Chronic Diseases 29:483-490.

CHAPTER 2
Mental Health Needs
of Asian Americans and Pacific Islanders

Joe Yamamoto, MD

Dr. Yamamoto's extensive clinical experience and his highly successful work as Director of the Asian/Pacific Counseling Service in Los Angeles render him particularly well qualified to comment on the mental health needs of Asian Americans and Pacific Islanders. As the paper below points out, there is a shortage of systematic data concerning the relationship of this population to the professional mental health service establishment; in spite of this, the need for culturally appropriate services has been demonstrated by clinics like Dr. Yamamoto's. The insights gained from this experience (such as the awareness of the role of stigma in preventing patients and their families from seeking needed care, mentioned below) thus deserve particular attention in research design and in service delivery.

The mental health needs of Asian Americans have been a matter of ongoing concern for some time; this concern is reflected in part in the report of the Task Panel on Special Populations of the President's Commission on Mental Health, and in the funding and subsequent work of the Pacific/Asian American Mental Health Research Center (P/AAMHRC). This Center and many concerned individuals have over the past ten years made progress toward clarifying these needs.

Some recent discussion in general psychiatry is relevant to the problem of ascertaining the needs of Asian Americans and Pacific Islanders. For example, Adler, Levinson, and Astrachan (1978) in their reexamination of the concept of prevention in mental health care, pointed out that there are four major categories of need in psychiatry: 1) medical, 2) rehabilitative, 3) social control, and 4) humanistic. Each of these areas has a corresponding set of "tasks." Arguing that concepts of prevention are most applicable to the medical and rehabilitative problems, the authors warn that "application of models of prevention in the social control and humanistic task areas has led to serious confusion." They go on to say:

. . . in the medical task area, efforts of primary prevention of mental illness remain very limited in scope and effectiveness. A commitment of research is important to efforts of primary prevention. Secondary prevention lies at the heart of the medical caring task, where early diagnosis and treatment are often of value. The work of rehabilitation lies both in the tertiary prevention of disease and in primary prevention of mental defect.

Their discussion points out the problems that can arise if public health concepts of prevention are applied to the tasks of psychiatry, especially if they are misapplied to the areas of social control and humanistic concerns.

With this exposition in mind, then, my effort herein will be to focus particularly on the two areas in which clinical prevention is a useful concept: medical and rehabilitative needs and tasks. Early diagnosis and clinical treatment are serious problems for Asian Americans and Pacific Islanders. This can be attributed to a complicated mix of factors, among which are: 1) Asian and Pacific Islander professional personnel are unevenly distributed among some of the ethnic groups; 2) because disorders are seldom diagnosed early due to the extreme stigma attached to mental illness by Asian and Pacific Islander groups, patients are not brought to treatment until the illness is advanced; 3) diagnosis may be inaccurate due to the lack of bilingual/bicultural personnel and the absence of diagnostic instruments in the appropriate languages; 4) very often, by the time the patients are seen they are seriously and chronically disordered, which complicates clinical treatment. Thus, prevention by means of early diagnosis and appropriate and adequate treatment has not been readily available to this group.

Evidence of the underutilization of mental health services by Asian Americans and Pacific Islanders is available from Honolulu, Seattle, San Francisco, and Los Angeles. In Los Angeles, for example, Asian Americans utilize only 40 percent of their proportion of mental health services. I believe that this low rate of utilization must be attributed not to a high level of mental health, but to the influence of stigma in preventing members of Asian and Pacific minority groups from seeking needed care. Estimates of the prevalence of psychiatric disorder in the general population vary, but a recent review of the literature on the psychiatric epidemiology of the United States by Regier, Goldberg, and Taube (1978) can provide a useful basis for comparison with what we know about Asian American patterns of mental health care utilization. These authors suggest that about fifteen percent of the population suffers from mental or emotional problems, but only three percent are seen by mental health professionals. They estimate that another nine percent are seen by general medical service people of one kind or another, and the remaining three percent never enter the professional health care system at all. Studies of this sort raise important questions regarding the rates and patterns of utilization of services by Asian Americans; extrapolating from the Los Angeles utilization data to the findings of Regier et al., it is evident that perhaps as few as 1.2 percent of Asian Americans who are in need of mental health care are receiving appropriate care.

It is apparent that we need more epidemiological data about the emotional health of Asian Americans and Pacific Islanders. Such data on the prevalence of disorders in the minority population should be compared with data on the rates and patterns of utilization of services, accounting for such things as the underrepresentation of Asians and Pacific Islanders in mental health facilities. When such data are available, they will make it possible to take appropriate steps to increase utilization and improve the quality of mental health services.

Once patients with incapacities have been diagnosed, emphasis shifts from the medical task to the rehabilitative task. In recent years there has been a general deemphasis on hospital care of the chronically psychotic, and most of these individuals have been discharged from hospital settings. Most are not receiving adequate care in the communities to which they have been discharged. Rehabilitation, then, must concentrate on minimizing the degree of impairment while maximizing coping abilities. There have been two exciting research reports concerning treatment of schizophrenic patients, which have important implications for research on the rehabilitation of Pacific/Asian American mental patients. Both papers address themselves to the issue of families and the schizophrenic patient. Goldstein et al. (1978) have found that relapses at six weeks and at six-month follow-up were least in patients who received both appropriate medication and family therapy, and most in those who received low doses of medication and no family therapy. The close family ties that are such an important feature in the life of most Asian Americans and Pacific Islanders could thus be a crucial factor in the development of appropriate therapies for chronic behavior disorders.

A second significant report by Vaughn and Leff (1976, supporting previous research by Brown et al.) reports on follow-up studies of discharged schizophrenic patients. Those who were returned to "highly emotional families" had a much greater tendency to relapse than those whose families were less expressive of emotion; this was found to be the case whether or not the patient remained on appropriate antipsychotic medication. Studies of this kind illustrate the important role of family life in the rehabilitation of mental patients, and suggest that similar research among Asian Americans would be of direct benefit to patients, families, and communities.

SUMMARY

In this brief outline I have attempted to touch on some issues and present some concerns that are important to the mental health of Asian Americans and Pacific Islanders. While avoiding the areas of social control and humanistic needs, I have suggested that several problems exist in the medical and rehabilitative areas. Our population suffers from a shortage of culturally appropriate professional services, and there is evidence to suggest that they tragically underutilize the services that are currently available. Until better epidemiological data is available, we must assume that Pacific/Asian Americans suffer from roughly the same amount of mental disorder as do other American populations, and we must do what we can to encourage greater utilization of services, the training of more bilingual/bicultural service providers, and the development of more appropriate diagnostic and therapeutic procedures in clinical treatment.

REFERENCES

Adler, David A., Daniel J. Levinson and Boris M. Astrachan
   1978 "The Concept of Prevention in Psychiatry." Archives of General Psychiatry 35:786-789 (June).

Goldstein, Michael J., Eliot H. Rodnick, Jerome R. Evans, Philip R. A. May and Mark R. Steinberg
   1978 "Drug and Family Therapy in the Aftercare of Acute Schizophrenics." Archives of General Psychiatry 35: 1169-1177 (October).

Regier, Darrel A., Irving D. Goldberg and Carl A. Taube
   1978 "The De Facto U.S. Mental Health Services System: A Public Health Perspective." Archives of General Psychiatry 35:685-693 (June).

Vaughn, Christine and Julian Leff
   1976 "The Measurement of Expressed Emotion in the Families of Psychiatric Patients." British Journal of Social and Clinical Psychology 15:157-165.

CHAPTER 3
Mental Health Delivery System to Asian Americans

Soon-Hyung Chung, MD

Dr. Chung is an experienced clinician with a predominantly Asian American clientele. One way in which she has attempted to overcome the stigma attached to the seeking of advice for mental health problems among Asian Americans has been to present a call-in television show in Honolulu. She was able to perform a valuable public education function with her show, while also responding to the specific needs of callers whose anonymity was safe in such a format. The recommendations Dr. Chung makes below reflect her experience with Asian/Pacific Americans and her sensitivity to the subtle barriers that prevent many of them from seeking needed care.

Although the United States has always been a country made up of many ethnic groups, only recently has this fact been acknowledged in the realization and implementation of mental health service delivery. Culturally appropriate services have been made available for America's ethnic minorities only in the last decade or two, and such services are still far from common for Asian Americans. There is, however, increasing official recognition that, in the words of Rosalynn Carter, cultural differences sometimes prevent certain minority groups from using mental health services. This concern is reflected in the report of the President's Commission on Mental Health (February 1978), which received 67 specific recommendations for improving services from the 25 members of the Subpanel on the Mental Health of Asian Pacific Americans. It is, however, clear that under today's economic conditions there are unlikely to be any major additions for Asian Americans to the government-funded mental health delivery system; thus our concern must be focused more on the currently available service delivery institutions, with an investigation of how they can be more adequately utilized for maximum effect in the interest of Asian/Pacific Americans.

This is especially crucial due to the rapid increase in the Asian American population since 1965, from 1.5 million in 1970 to an estimated 3 million in 1980. The needs of recent immigrants and refugees will have to be considered carefully as well.

Although the problems that confront Asian Americans and Pacific Islanders in obtaining adequate mental health care are in many respects not too different from those of any disadvantaged minority, they seem to be exaggerated in extent and magnitude by language barriers and by the cultural heterogeneity of Asian/Pacific groups. It can also be argued that the closely intertwined community life of some Asian American groups is a complicating factor for individuals and families in need of mental health services.

Major factors within the existing mental health delivery system that negatively affect Asian Americans are itemized below:

1) Staff people who deal with Asian/Pacific Americans tend to be unfamiliar with and insensitive to their culture and acculturation situations and ethnic characteristics.

2) Discrimination against Asian Americans often amounts to institutional racism, but it is seldom perceived as such.

3) There is a shortage of bilingual and/or bicultural personnel who can provide more appropriate and sensitive services to Pacific/Asian Americans.

4) Currently existing programs that have been serving Asian and Pacific Americans are afflicted with severe and increasing financial limitations.

5) Very little has been attempted within the organized mental health care delivery system in the way of providing culturally relevant service modalities; the resources of folk and traditional healers are not utilized at all, and there are almost no outreach programs designed to educate the Asian/Pacific communities regarding the services that are available to them through the conventional channels.

6) Existing mental health services are poorly integrated with Asian American community services such as youth programs, family counseling, child welfare, and services to the elderly and handicapped.

7) There is a lack of liaison between other Asian American community organizations (of which there are many wherever there is an established community) and public mental health and social service agencies.

8) In many cases, rigid definitions of catchment areas and distribution of publically available services prevent Asian Americans from seeking ethno-culturally appropriate services even in cities where they are available.

9) The system fails to utilize many bilingual and bicultural Asian and Pacific Islander service providers due to overly strict licensure and training requirements. (New immigrant and refugee groups are especially affected by this problem, as in many cases members of these ethnic groups have not had the opportunity to acquire the specialized training required to meet state licensing requirements.)

10) In many Asian/Pacific communities, a strong stigma is attached to behavior problems and to the notion of mental illness. This can prevent many who are in need of care from seeking it, especially if they fear being "shamed" in the close-knit ethnic communities of which they are likely to be a part. Mass media outreach programs in various Asian languages can be one solution to this difficult problem.

11) Asian Americans are allowed very little participation in planning and decision-making processes that affect mental health service programs.

12) Continuing education programs that could heighten the awareness among non-Asian/Pacific service providers of Asian American cultural differences and needs are in general not available.

13) There is almost no form of mental health service that can help Asian Americans who are in acute crisis or who are isolated from cohesive ethnic enclaves (such as Asian American wives of U.S. servicemen). A nation- or state-wide hotline service in appropriate languages might be an inexpensive way to partially meet this need.

CHAPTER 4
Manpower Training and Licensing Problems Facing Asian Americans Entering the Health Field

Jane F. Lee, MD

Dr. Lee's detailed report on licensing and manpower training is based on her experience as a member of California's Board of Medical Quality Assurance and as a family practitioner and acupuncturist in the Bay Area. Some of the summary tables and statute citations have been abstracted herein to save space, but even in its shortened form this paper makes very clear the obstacles facing Asian Americans who wish to enter the health professions. Some of these obstacles will have to be eliminated if the Asian Pacific community is ever to have an adequate pool of service providers of appropriate linguistic and cultural backgrounds.

In order to study the manpower training and licensing problems facing Asian Americans, it is necessary to look briefly at our historical background and population characteristics. Generally speaking, the term "Asian American" includes Chinese, Japanese, Koreans, Filipinos, South and Southeast Asian peoples, and Pacific Islanders (for example, Samoans and Guamanians).

HISTORY

The migrations of Asians to the U.S. began in the mid-1800s with the arrival of the Chinese in California. Between 1850 and 1900, the early Chinese immigrants were first welcomed, later tolerated, and finally legally excluded as a result of political pressure on the part of California labor interests. Chinese laborers were not only barred from entering this country by the Chinese exclusion acts of 1882, 1892, and 1902, but those already residing in the U.S. were denied citizenship; the Quota Act of 1924 even excluded Chinese wives of American citizens. The economic activities of the Chinese were thus shifted from competitive fields to less desirable occupations such as personal service. In 1943, the ban on Chinese immigration was lifted to allow entry of an annual quota of 100, and in 1945 the War Brides Act allowed entry of 6,000

Chinese women. With the Immigration and Nationality Act of 1965, the annual quota for immigrants was set on a world-wide basis, allowing 170,000 people per year from the eastern hemisphere (20,000 for each foreign state). In 1968, the National Origins Quota Act was finally repealed altogether, and since that time there has been a yearly increase in the number of Chinese admitted to the U.S., averaging 18,000 annually since 1965. The early development of Chinatowns in major urban centers, to which many subsequent immigrants were attracted, was a response to prejudice and discrimination in the wider American community.

Japanese migrants began to arrive in the U.S. in the late 1890s. Many of the first wave of Japanese immigration remained in the sugar-cane fields of Hawaii, but shortly thereafter many came to the continental United States and Canada, settling mainly on the West Coast.

Filipinos did not immigrate in any numbers until 1924, whereupon they settled mainly in Hawaii and the two seaboards of the U.S. Like other Asian American groups, since 1965 this early wave of Filipino immigrants has been supplemented by a new and numerous group that is socially and historically quite distinct from their Filipino American predecessors.

Citizenship to first generation Asians was denied until December 1943 for the Chinese, July 1946 for Filipinos, and December 1952 for the Japanese. The denial of citizenship and consequent threat of deportation, denial of the right to own property, incarceration in concentration camps, and the exclusion and immigration quota acts, have led to a fear of government and a strong sense of powerlessness that has alienated Asian Americans from the larger U.S. society.

The 1970 Census enumerated about 1.5 million Asian Americans, and the partial census of 1977 estimated that the Asian American population had risen to two million. These findings probably constitute an underenumeration; large segments of the Asian community were not reached or did not respond to the census out of suspicion or English illiteracy. In addition, 200,000 persons of South and Southeast Asian ancestry were excluded from the census categories cited. It is projected that by 1980 Asian Americans will exceed three million, and that the Filipinos, closely followed by the Chinese, will overtake the Japanese in population.

Geographic distribution breakdowns show that 90 percent of Asian Americans are in major metropolitan areas, predominantly in Hawaii, California, New York, Washington, Illinois, and Massachusetts. Although they comprise only two percent of the population nationwide, in certain cities of the West Coast and Northeast the percentage is much higher; thus, Asian Americans comprise 13 percent of the population of San Francisco, 3 percent in Los

Angeles/Long Beach, and 85 percent in Honolulu. Recent immigration increases will no doubt increase the overall percentage as well as the higher local percentages in some metropolitan areas. From 1930 to 1970, the percentage of professional workers in the United States has risen from 1 percent to 21 percent. Foreign-born professionals, however, have not benefited equally from this expansion of professional opportunities. Language difficulties, problems of acculturation, and discrimination have restricted their participation in the higher levels of occupational achievement. Important barriers to professional occupations are faced by native-born Asian Americans as well, but it is the foreign-born and especially the foreign-trained for whom most barriers have been raised.

MANPOWER TRAINING

Among the health fields, the greatest restrictions encountered by Asian Americans are in medicine, dentistry, nursing, and pharmacy. These are also the professional areas listed by the Immigration and Naturalization Service (1976) as being in shortest supply, and therefore having highest priority for admission to permanent residency. In the period from 1967 to 1976, 47 percent of nurses, 63.8 percent of dentists, 77.1 percent of pharmacists, and 61.0 percent of physicians admitted from all foreign countries were from Asia. This sizeable group of professional Asian immigrants has been prevented by licensing requirements from entering the pool of available medical service personnel in comparable numbers, however.

Selection of Asian Americans for entrance into health professional schools has been discriminatory in some respects. In general, U.S. population quotas have been used as the basis for selection of Asian Americans where minority quota systems are in use. In the case of the Chinese, for example, California colleges use the percentage of Chinese in the total population (0.5 percent) as their guide in selecting entering classes, ignoring the greater need for Chinese professionals in California where the Chinese proportion of the population greatly exceeds the national percentage. The U.S. Supreme Court's recent decision regarding minority admissions programs in the Bakke vs. University of California case is a substantial setback for minority students seeking admission to health professional schools. The court held that the University of California, Davis, Medical School discriminated against white applicants by reserving 16 places for minority students; it ruled that colleges and universities could consider race and ethnicity in admissions programs as long as they did not use numerical quotas. Currently Asians occupy a slightly higher percentage of the available space in the health professional schools than their overall percentage of the national population. But in this case "Asian" almost inevitably refers to Chinese and Japanese students, leaving a radical imbalance in the training of health professionals from the other Asian American ethnic groups. It thus seems unlikely that the comparative shortage of Asian Americans in the health professions will be remedied in the near future if we depend only upon U.S. professional schools to provide the needed well-trained personnel. It is important to note the heterogeneity of the Asian American population. Not only do the foreign-born differ markedly from the American-born, but first-generation Asian Americans differ from the second and third generations, which in some respects differ in turn from each other. In addition, each of the ethnic groups (Chinese, Japanese, Filipino, Sri Lankan, etc.) is unique in its language and culture, taking pride in its distinct traditions. It is not surprising, then, that many Pacific/Asian Americans prefer to travel a great distance to obtain health care from a bilingual or bicultural professional whom they perceive to be sympathetic rather than going to a closer facility with no ethnically identifiable personnel.

In this respect Pacific Islanders face an especially acute problem, since there are very few professional health providers from these ethnic groups. At present there are next to no Samoan or Guamanian physicians, psychologists, or psychiatrists.

Bilingualism and biculturalism should be encouraged in manpower training policy, enabling Asian Americans to compete equally with other Americans for health service jobs while permitting Asian and Pacific ethnic groups to preserve their own customs and community lifestyles. Asian American health manpower is at present inadequate to properly serve America's Asian and Pacific ethnic communities.

LAWS AND EXAMINATIONS PERTAINING TO FOREIGN MEDICAL GRADUATES

Foreign medical graduates (FMGs) have in recent years been perceived as a special social problem in the United States. Various laws requiring special assessment procedures prior to licensing them to practice have been passed, among them the Health Professions Education Assistance Act (October 1976) and amendments to the Immigration and Nationality Act affecting the entry of alien physicians to the U.S. (1977). These removed physicians, pharmacists, and nurses from the Immigration Service's list of most-needed professions, and imposed restrictions on the entry of foreign physicians to the United States for the purpose of receiving graduate medical training. They also exempted from these restrictions alien physicians "who are of national or international renown in the field of medicine." The Asian/Pacific subcommittee of the President's Commission on Mental Health found these laws to have racist implications. The subcommittee recommended that Asian/

Pacific foreign medical graduates already in this country be provided with orientation programs that would prepare them for licensing and specialty training. They based their recommendation on their finding that foreign medical graduates are unfairly limited in their access to high quality training institutions and academic centers.

Current or proposed examinations for FMG's are as follows:

Education Commission for Foreign Medical Graduates (ECFMG): The goal of the ECFMG exam has been to verify the credentials and evaluate the educational qualifications of foreign medical graduates who wish to advance their training in the United States. This examination applies only to FMGs, not to graduates of U.S. medical schools, and 45 of the 50 states require that FMGs pass before they can be licensed to practice or enter graduate training programs--i.e., internships and residencies. This exam makes it unnecessary to develop any form of accreditation for medical training systems in other parts of the world (about 700 medical schools in more than 120 countries). Results of this test have confirmed the fact that medical training is extremely variable from country to country.

Visa Qualifying Examination (VQE): This exam has been adopted by the Department of Health, Education, and Welfare as an equivalency assessment to be used where Parts I and II of the National Board exams have not been taken. Alien physicians must meet the English requirements of the ECFMG before taking this two-day examination. The VQE will be given annually, but a high failure rate is expected since its contents are oriented to American medical school curricula.

Comprehensive Qualifying Examination (CQE): A comprehensive qualifying exam is now being considered as a prerequisite to entering graduate medical education programs in this country. The CQE would be required of all candidates, foreign and U.S. graduates alike.

Federation Licensing Examination (FLEX): This is the state licensing examination given each year to all medical graduates except those who receive state licensure by endorsement of their National Board after they have taken Board exams.

Some states have enacted special regulations regarding the licensure of FMGs to practice medicine. In California, for example, the Board of Medical Quality Assurance (under the Department of Consumer Affairs) has developed special requirements for the many foreign medical graduates who have settled in that state. These requirements include longer postgraduate clinical experience than is required of U.S. medical graduates, and an additional oral clinical examination beyond the FLEX exam which is required of all candidates for licensure. Special certificates can be issued to physicians holding faculty positions in medical schools who are not actively engaged in clinical practice. FMGs who are accepted into approved postgraduate training programs in California may also be temporarily certified to participate in clinical programs of their departments until the program is completed and they are eligible for full licensure. These provisions are relatively liberal but they are exclusively oriented to graduates of medical training systems that closely resemble those of the United States.

Licensing of FMGs in the state of New York differs from that for U.S. medical graduates only in that the candidate's medical school must be listed in the World Directory of Medical Schools and in that he/she must pass the ECFMG examination. All candidates for licensure must have postgraduate hospital training in the U.S and must pass the FLEX exam. Postgraduate training in foreign hospitals and medical schools is not considered adequate or equivalent for licensure in New York.

The regulations of other states are extremely various but in almost all cases require that FMGs have additional training beyond that required for U.S. graduates. The use of the FLEX exam by all 50 states has somewhat facilitated the licensing of FMGs; as a result, in more than half the states it is possible to substitute foreign postgraduate training for a U.S. internship.

In many cases requirements of foreign candidates for licensure in the fields of dentistry and pharmacy have been even more strict than those for physicians. Not only has U.S. postgraduate education been required, but further years of basic undergraduate education have often been necessary for these practitioners. Some of these provisions have recently been liberalized, and credit and evaluation services may occasionally be employed to determine equivalency in the foreign training program.

Most states have no restriction barring foreign-trained nurses from applying for nursing license examinations, although a few states require citizenship. In a majority of states foreign nurses may even practice and be licensed without having to pass qualifying exams, providing their training is satisfactory to the state board of nursing.

BARRIERS TO ASIAN AMERICANS
IN THE HEALTH PROFESSIONS

As pointed out earlier, the migration of highly trained health professionals from Asian countries to the United States has increased dramatically since 1965. Dreams of successful careers in the specialties for which they were trained have faded as these immigrants have realized that the quality of the education they received in their native lands is generally considered to be inferior to that which is available in the U.S. For many of these individuals, competition for postgraduate training positions has made it nearly impossible to upgrade their skills to levels required by licensing boards. At best, long years of further study and financial sacrifice are required before the foreign-trained can hope to participate appropriately in America's health care system.

This is not a problem solely for the professionals themselves. It may well be a factor in Asian American underutilization of services, as there is a shortage of health care providers who are sensitive to the traditions, values, and attitudes of America's Asian ethnics. In a study of health care for minority patients, E. H. White notes that an increase in the number of Asian health professionals would help to increase such sensitivity to the specific needs of minority patients.

For those foreign professionals who have not been able to meet the requirements discussed above, unemployment or underemployment has been their fate. Few studies have been made that have followed the individual careers of foreign health professionals. A study done in the state of Washington indicates, however, that of the foreign medical graduates sampled, their years of training were comparable to those of their U.S. counterparts in 80-85 percent of the cases; 87 percent of the FMGs had been licensed to practice in their respective home countries. Although 44 percent of them had had further professional education in the U.S., only 69.2 percent had found employment in their own health profession, and not all of these were practicing at the professional level for which they had been trained, many having to settle for work as technicians or paraprofessionals due to licensing difficulties. Furthermore, 64 percent of the sample had no license of any kind.

One problem that seems to affect the success of FMGs in becoming licensed is inexperience with standardized tests. Those who are able to take the necessary examinations several times benefit from an improved passing rate for repeaters. This improved pass rate may reflect not only experience in answering multiple choice-type questions, but also increasing English skills as time in this country lengthens. The fact that even short-term professional education in the U.S. also significantly improves pass rates may have more to do with increasing English skills than with improved clinical skills.

Six recommendations may be made regarding the situation of Asian Americans in the health professions:

1) An intense refresher course should be provided to assist Asian-educated doctors, nurses, pharmacists, and dentists to pass licensing examinations.

2) These should be supplemented with remedial English classes that provide training in standardized test-taking.

3) Existing licensing laws should be changed to work less hardship on the qualified health professionals from other countries who are being prevented from working in their chosen specialties.

4) A continual effort should be made to provide hospital internship and residency opportunities for foreign medical graduates who have passed the ECFMG. At present, competition for this type of post-graduate training is so great that most FMGs are forced to take hospital staff positions that provide a minimum of training and supervision.

5) Asian Americans should classify as minorities for such things as medical school admissions programs and financial aid.

6) Asian Americans should be brought into full participation in America's social, political, and economic life.

CONCLUSIONS

Studies of American-trained and foreign-trained Asian Americans have shown that there is considerable diversity in the cultural traits, degree of acculturation, and ethnic consciousness of these two groups. Within each of the two groups there are also great differences in ethnic composition. The greater the degree of acculturation of Asian health professionals, the easier it is for them to overcome the social, legal, and economic barriers facing them. Health manpower studies indicate a greater need of Asian Americans in most of the health fields. A failure to accord Asian Americans consideration as minorities for acceptance into health careers leads to a shortage of students to fill this need. Secondly, licensing restrictions, especially in dentistry and pharmacy, have limited foreign graduates in particular in these fields. American-born Asian Americans, once educated, have had little difficulty in obtaining licenses in their respective specialties. However, upward mobility and advancement in status are still slowed by prejudiced treatment given to Asian Americans, as well as by their relative lack of involvement in American political life.

CHAPTER 5
National Health Insurance

Hernan M. Reyes, MD

Among the many controversies that surround the problem
of national health insurance is the legitimate concern of
America's ethnic minorities that their special needs
should not be submerged in any large-scale program that
ignores such factors as ethnic and linguistic differences.
Dr. Reyes' original paper discussed the two major proposed programs at the time of the Task Force meeting
from the point of view of Pacific/Asian Americans; here
it has been edited somewhat to highlight the issues that
are raised by any national health insurance plan, rather
than the details of specific proposed legislation. A series
of recommendations are made regarding the basic
requirements that any plan should meet, with emphasis
not only on the needs of Asian Americans and Pacific
Islanders, but also on the provision of good health care to
all Americans regardless of their ethnicity.

The Asian/Pacific American community numbers about three
million individuals, including Chinese, Japanese, Filipino, Korean,
Indian, Pakistani, Cambodian, Laotian, Vietnamese, Hawaiian,
Guamanian, and Samoan groups. Ninety percent of them reside in
the metropolitan areas of Los Angeles, San Francisco, Honolulu,
Chicago, and New York.

Asian/Pacific Islanders are often perceived as a "model minority," an immigrant group that has "made it" in American society.
This is absolutely a myth. Discrimination exists in the form of a
lack of opportunity in education, employment, housing, and health
and social service delivery. Health-related problems, and the
delivery of health care, are complicated for many Pacific/Asian
Americans by low socioeconomic status, inadequate information on
the availability of health care services, inadequate knowledge of
health problems inherent to Asians on the part of health care providers, language barriers, and cultural attitudes that in many cases
prevent the seeking of professional attention until later stages of
disease.

Inadequate education and resources foster a lack of concern for preventive medicine in the public and among health care professionals, especially since medical emphasis has always been on the treatment and cure of disease, rather than on its prevention. This is one of the fundamental problems that must be considered in the design of a national health insurance program. Several such programs are currently being considered by the President, Congress, and private industry. Since the Asian/Pacific American is as vulnerable as any other minority group member to the provisions of whatever form of national health insurance is finally provided, it is important to evaluate the options from this minority perspective.

Any acceptable form of national health insurance should attain three main goals:

1) To remove inequalities in access to health care.

2) To alleviate the burden on individuals of excessive medical expenses.

3) To control the overall cost of health care, which has escalated dramatically during recent years. (Estimated spending by the health industry is currently one hundred billion dollars per year.)

There are currently three groups of people for whom total national health insurance coverage is absolutely mandatory. They are the aged, the poor, and the working poor whose incomes are very near the poverty level, and whose insurance premiums may represent as much as 20 percent of their take-home pay.

While it is true that there are health care services delivered to the first two groups through medicare and medicaid, experience with these two systems has shown numerous frustrating deficiencies and shortcomings. Medicare covers only about 70 percent of the cost of health care for the elderly, while medicaid benefits and eligibility vary from state to state, with abuses by patients and providers. The total health care that is provided by adequate health insurance is outside the reach of the working poor, whose whole family income is threatened by any illness.

Two contrasting types of national health insurance have been proposed in Congress. Senator Kennedy's plan would establish a national health insurance program covering the entire population, and providing a range of health services with no payment required of the patient. The program would be financed by a federal payroll tax on employers and employees, a tax on unearned income, and on federal general revenues. The proposal includes provisions designed to reorganize the delivery of health services, improve health planning, and increase the supply of health care manpower facilities.

Alternative plans have advocated less government involvement in health care delivery, with more dependence on private insurance plans and private medical services. For example, a House bill introduced by Representative Tim Lee Carter of Kentucky called for a three-part national program, including:

1) An employee health care benefit program requiring employers to offer private health insurance to their employees.

2) A state-assisted health center program providing coverage for low income families, and for families in employment groups who are high medical risks for health insurance.

3) A federal health care program for the aged, representing in effect an expanded medicare program.

All three of the programs under this plan would offer the same range of medical services and protect their beneficiaries against the cost of catastrophic illness. State governments would have major responsibility for supervision of employee programs and administration of the state-assisted health insurance, as well as for the regulation of insurance carriers and health services providers. Federal guidelines would be followed by the states in these activities.

In July of 1978, President Carter established ten principles as the basis of his national health insurance plan. These are as follows:

1) "The plan should assure that all Americans have comprehensive health care coverage, including protection against catastrophic medical expenses."

2) Quality health care should be available to all.

3) Americans should have "freedom of choice in the selection of physicians, hospitals, and health delivery systems."

4) Unnecessary health care spending must be reduced with aggressive cost containment and strengthening of the "competitive forces in the health care sector."

5) Additional public and private expenditures should be "substantially offset by savings from greater efficiency."

6) There is to be no additional federal spending until fiscal year 1983, and "the plan should be phased in gradually" with consideration given to economic and administrative adjustments as the plan moves from phase to phase. "The experience of other government pro- grams, in which expenditure far exceeded initial projections, must not be repeated."

7) The plan would be financed through government funding and contributions from both employers and employees, with careful consideration given to the "ability of many consumers to share a moderate portion of the cost of their care."

8) "A significant role" would be reserved for the private insurance industry under government regulation.

9) The plan should promote "ambulatory and preventive services, attracting personnel to underserved rural and urban areas and encouraging the use of prepaid health plans."

10) "The plan should assure consumer representation throughout its operation."

President Carter's health principles, if they can be properly implemented and adequately established, would in essence fill the health care needs of all Americans. But principles are not programs, and certain problems in the implementation of any national health program must be considered.

The experience of the British National Health Service is an important example for study. Legislation to prevent the pitfalls of full government financing of total care for the entire population must be seriously considered. In the words of an editorial from the Chicago Tribune (July 26, 1978):

. . . the British are paying a heavy price--in inconvenience, high taxes, long waits, and in some cases dangerously poor care--for their medical system. But so great is the lure of any free service that it seems unlikely they will agree to any basic changes.

Whatever form of national health insurance legislation is eventually enacted, certain basic requirements must be met to satisfy the needs of Pacific/Asian Americans. Anyone living in the United States should be eligible for coverage, regardless of whether he is a citizen, resident-alien, or visitor. There should be no restrictions whatsoever to the ready availability of medical care to anyone who needs it. Furthermore, education programs in appropriate languages must be undertaken to disseminate health system information to new immigrants of Asian-Pacific origin, who in most instances are not aware of their rights and privileges.

A new and fundamental emphasis on prevention must be adopted if the spiralling costs of health care are to be controlled. Among other steps in this direction, programs of public health education (multilingual) should be accompanied by education of health service personnel regarding diseases endemic in Asian and Pacific areas. Immunization, environmental evaluation, and periodic diagnostic and screening examinations should focus particularly on the medical needs of minority and immigrant groups as well as on those of the poor and the aged.

The range of personal medical services should include dental, home, and nursing care, rehabilitation, drugs, appliances, and a full range of mental health services. There should be no regulation or restriction of these benefits.

Health care resources will have to be increased in certain service sectors: there will have to be more outpatient clinics, mental health clinics, and neighborhood health centers, staffed with adequate medical and paramedical personnel. The medical school curriculum may need to be restructured to train more family health practitioners and to include health care education in all levels of the medical training system.

Provision must be made for adequate bilingual treatment and education programs, such that language need not be a barrier to receiving good health care under any health insurance plan. Proper distribution of a full range of health care personnel should be provided for, with special emphasis on rural and inner-city areas, Native American communities, areas of minority and immigrant concentration, and migrant labor camps.

Strong regulation of any national health insurance plan is essential to prevent abuse of services and to maximize public health effectiveness. A federal commission should be empowered to continually investigate, formulate, and enforce cost control measures. The formula for financing national health insurance should combine employer contributions (even up to 75 percent of premium amount), minimal employee contributions, increased social security withholding, and general revenue contributions. The last source of income would finance health services to the poor, the aged, the unemployed, and the disabled.

A national health commission which represents the government, medical care providers, and consumers should be responsible for mediating the problems which arise as the national health insurance plan is implemented and evolved. This commission must examine the needs of every segment of society, making sure that cost control is exercised by eliminating unnecessary expenses, providing for effective preventive medicine, and administering the plan in order to achieve all the goals set forth and to guarantee decent health care for every American.

CHAPTER 6
Pacific/Asian Culture and Experience in Health and Illness: Report of a Planning Committee

Joe Okimoto, MD, and Anthony Ishisaka

The following outline resulted from the convening of a committee to plan a symposium on the topic of Pacific/Asian American Culture and Experience in Health and Illness. Committee members included Joe Okimoto and Tony Ishisaka, co-chairpersons; Dorothy Cordova; Arthur Kleinman; Min Masuda; Betty Mitsunaga; Stanley Sue; Keh-Ming Lin; and Eugene Ko. Out of their considerable collective experience in research in Asian and Pacific communities, and in service delivery to such communities, this group compiled the program below. Although funds have not yet been raised for such a symposium, the proposed topics represent areas in which important research is now being done. They are, furthermore, areas in which much further research needs to be done, and in which a deeper understanding of sociocultural conditions would be a contribution not only to policy makers but to all Pacific/Asian Americans and to the general study of health and health care.

I. Pacific/Asian Culture, Health, and Illness
    The Impact of Culture on the Presentation of Illness
    Health Perceptions and Beliefs Among Asians
    Somatization
    The Immigrant Experience

II. Epidemiologic Studies Among Pacific/Asian Groups
    Chronic Disease in Asians
    Illness Among Chinese
    The Chinese Experience and Health Status
    Socioeconomic Factors in Health Status among
        Pacific/Asians
    Psychiatric Epidemiology

III. Pacific/Asian Therapeutic Practices and Institutions
    Asian Health Maintenance Practices and Institutions
    Cultural Aspects of Psychotherapy
    Acupuncture and Other "Folk Medicine"
    Pathways to Health Care
    Morita Therapy and Asian Americans
    Counseling of Asian Americans

IV.   The Delivery of Health and Mental Health Services
           Utilization of Mental Health Services by Asians
           Impact of Language Differences on Health Care Delivery
           Racism and Health Care Delivery
           Health Manpower and Health Services to Pacific/Asians
           The Blend of Old and New Health Care - Lessons from
               China
           Health Care for Immigrant Children

V.   Psychopharmacology with Asians

VI.   Special Topics
           Pacific/Asian Youth, Drug and Alcohol Abuse, Juvenile
               Delinquency and Academic Dropouts
           Suicide Among Pacific/Asians
           Acculturation and Identity in Pacific/Asian Groups
           Education for Improved Health Services

Appendix

Holistic Health: A Public Policy Report on a Meeting
Sponsored by the East West Academy of Healing Arts
(Washington, D.C., April, 1978)

Judith Farquhar

The report below was considered to be of interest to the
health and mental health task force as a way of providing
some information on the context of national health
reform within which Asian/Pacific Americans may be able
to make their special voice heard. The meeting concerned was the first national policy meeting to bring
together many of the health reform activists who have
concerned themselves with the somewhat vaguely defined
notion of "holistic health." It is significant for the
purposes of the task force that this concept is strongly
associated with Asian culture, and that the meeting
sponsor was an organization committed to productive
exchange and synthesis between Asian and American
healing systems. If we take seriously the idea of
integrating alternative therapies into the American
medical care system, it is organizations such as the East
West Academy of Healing Arts (and its director Effie Poy
Yew Chow) to which we can turn for specific guidance.
Multicultural and heterogeneous networks of reform-
oriented people such as the one assembled for this
meeting may turn out to be an important constituency for
Asian Americans in their efforts to achieve more appropriate health and mental health care. These considerations led to our submitting a report on the meeting to the
task force and to our reprinting it here as an appendix.

The meeting participants represented a wide range of interests
and came from many professional backgrounds. The enthusiasm
with which the extremely varied program was received indicated
that the holistic health movement may be able to encompass many
health reform groups in the U.S. If such a community of interests is
to become a political coalition, it seems important to summarize
and examine concerns addressed at the meeting in terms of their
implications and potential social impact.

The issues that concerned most meeting participants can be grouped under three main headings: 1) the inadequacies of currently dominant models of medical practice; 2) multiculturalism; and 3) preventive medicine, self-care, and "wellness."

THE INADEQUACIES OF CURRENTLY DOMINANT MODELS OF MEDICAL PRACTICE

Dr. Lythcott, assistant surgeon general and administrator of the Health Services Administration of DHEW, pointed out that the spectacular success of conventional Western medicine in combatting infectious diseases has not been matched by a comparable success in dealing with chronic conditions. He also noted that the costs of chronic disease treatment are rising beyond our capacity to support them, and that preventive medicine and health maintenance programs must be the focus of public policy in the future.

California assemblyman Vasconcellos cited the traditional "mystification" and hierarchical structure of the medical profession, and mentioned trends toward self-care and universal education as positive developments in health care reform.

Dr. Lee, a family practitioner and acupuncturist, described the advantages of nonintrusive therapies such as acupuncture, and scored the conservatism of licensing boards and medical organizations in opposing their positive and well-monitored use.

Psychologist Alberto Villoldo emphasized the way in which traditional Latino healing involved the whole community in a kind of life-style adjustment, and advocated movement away from the mentalist bias in psychotherapy in dealing with many ethnic clients.

Dr. Jerome Frank of Johns Hopkins University pointed out that holistic healing has "snuc____ ___" Western medicine under the name of the placebo effect. _____ research has done little to understand processes in healing that do not fall into the conventional therapeutic categories; he suggested that faith in the healer may be a major factor in all therapies.

Native American healer Oh Shinnah Fastwolf believes that our civilization has been foolishly denying the vital link between human life and the health of "Our Earth Mother." She urged attention to the spiritual aspects of health as an essential part of holistic healing.

Nutritionist Dr. Sheldon Margen expressed his concern that as our diet becomes more specialized and industrialized and as the ecological niche of our species becomes smaller, we become less flexible and more dependent. He believes that the way to more heathful nutrition involves more public involvement in policy relating to food production and marketing.

Dr. Kenneth Greenspan, researcher in biofeedback and stress-related disorders, pointed out that many of the new therapies of the holistic health movement run counter to the traditionally objective viewpoint of professional medicine. Health care professionals must learn to adopt a more subjective orientation in order to be effective in these new treatment modalities.

Naturopath Jack Schwarz stated that we are less effective than we could be in controlling our own states of health, and that we have been the victims of a belief system that encourages us to be passive about self-healing.

Dr. Lowell Levin, Yale Professor of Public Health, pointed out that medical practice in the United States has traditionally operated with narrow professional assumptions, many of which are not borne out by the facts. Among the many problematic assumptions he listed was the treatment of health as a commodity, resulting in the ideas that health reform consists in getting more professional medical care to more people and that there should be a service for every need and a need for every service. He outlined and refuted three components of what he called the professional health fantasy: 1) improvements in health care over the last century have been due to the actions of health care professionals. In fact, only 3.5% of the decline in mortality since the late nineteenth century can be reasonably attributed to professional medical activities. Improved public health measures have played a much larger role. 2) When medical care has an effect it is a beneficial one. Dr. Levin pointed out that iatrogenic (physician-related) effects are on the rise, and, depending upon how the category is defined, could be seen to have reached epidemic proportions. 3) Most health care is provided by medical professionals. This assumption fails to take account of self-care which constitutes 75% of all acute health care and nearly 100% of all preventive care. Dr. Levin noted important shifts within professional medicine, for example the shift from cure to care as the ratio of chronic to acute disorders has dramatically risen. There is an increased recognition of the role of life-style in many chronic conditions, as well, and consumer activism has led to a new economic and bureaucratic model of medical practice to replace the old "family doctor" medical model. He also pointed out that many social problems such as child abuse and alcoholism have been "medicalized." These changes have their positive and negative sides, and Dr. Levin sees the increasing interest in a wide variety of self-help procedures and organizations as the most positive addition to the contemporary health care scene.

Urban planner William Milliken expressed his concern about the large dehumanizing institutions of contemporary health care delivery and urged an end to the paternalism in provider-client relationships.

Participants in a workshop on research in holistic health methods explored ways of systematizing subjective data from new clinical methods, as well as policy issues such as the legalization of certain FDA-prohibited substances. The advantages of legalizing such drugs as Laetrile were balanced by a serious caution about bringing back the days of uncontrolled exploitation of the sick with worthless patent medicines. Other research problems were discussed, such as the methodological problems of comparing individual clinical indices with standardized statistical curves, and development of an "individual health profile" was urged. It was also pointed out that research on aspects of preventive medicine has been hindered by the absence of any measures of normality or "wellness."

MULTICULTURALISM

There were representatives of a variety of healing traditions at the meeting, and the emphasis was on participants learning from each other. Effie Poy Yew Chow of the East West Academy of Healing Arts (the chief conference organizer) emphasized the fundamental commonalities of all major world medical systems, and gave a crowd-pleasing demonstration of ch'i meridians, or energy pathways, used in Chinese therapies.

In a multicultural panel discussion, Jane Lee discussed the holism of Chinese medicine, explaining that the Western mind-body dichotomy did not prevail in Asian systems. She listed a variety of Chinese therapies that have long histories of clinical efficacy and cost-effectiveness.

Alberto Villoldo spoke about the mode of psychotherapy that he had developed in an effort to be sensitive to the culture and conditions of his Latino clients. Not only is it important to treat the whole life-style and "communal" self, but the therapist must also be able to help minority individuals break out of the "cultural trance" of poverty and discrimination in order to develop their full potential as human beings. He felt that, to this end, the health care professions need a definition of "the optimal human being."

Beverly Robinson, UCLA professor of folklore, talked about the basic premises of Afro-American healing beliefs, emphasizing their spiritual nature and the importance of the idea that "with faith, all things are possible." She stated that need, economic considerations, and cultural appropriateness all affect the way in which health care is handled in the black community.

Oh Shinnah Fastwolf felt that spiritual considerations and harmony with the cosmos are important for the health of all peoples and that no true health is possible for humans apart from the total well-being of the planet.

The many half-day workshops on these and other "untraditional" therapies (from the viewpoint of Western medicine) explored the characteristics and implications of such healing systems, with a special emphasis on their relevance to health care reform at the policy and implementation levels.

PREVENTIVE MEDICINE, SELF-CARE, "WELLNESS"

There was general agreement at the conference that preventive care will have to occupy a much larger place in the health care systems of the future, for reasons of cost-effectiveness and because so much of medical care has shifted to the treatment of life-style related conditions such as cardiovascular disease and many forms of cancer. The concept of preventive care articulates with parallel interests in self-care and "high level wellness," and raises many issues concerning the relationship between health policy and individual responsibility.

Some participants emphasized the continuum between the traditional spheres of medical activity and chronic social problems such as alcoholism and drug abuse. As attention shifts to "treatment of the whole person," it will become harder to distinguish the proper sphere of medicine from that of much wider issues of social policy.

Many speakers were primarily concerned with the normative and evaluative dimensions of such a trend. Mr. Vasconcellos, for example, mentioned four directions in which he sees contemporary health care progressing: 1) toward demystification of the traditional authority structures in medicine, accompanied by 2) a related horizontal movement toward democratization of health care, involving such movements as self-care and the growing paraprofessional fields; 3) toward individualization, that is, an increasing interest in adapting medical activities to the needs of the individual; and 4) toward personalization, or an emphasis on the full development of persons within the framework of human potential and liberation movements. He saw these as positive and irreversible historical trends in American society, leading to what he called "a radical redefinition of what it means to be human." Along with some of the other speakers and many participants, he saw various forms of negative attitude as a major part of the fragmentation and "dichotomization" of modern life, and advocated a return to the state of "original innocence" that characterizes human life and health when it is not subjected to such destructive factors.

Speakers such as Ms. Chow and Mr. Schwarz offered experiential viewpoints on the powers of self-control of bodily states as an aspect of preventive self-care, and Dr. Levin pointed out the social significance of the many effective self-care movements now active in the U.S. There were more specifically clinical points made about self-care as well. Jane Lee demonstrated in her workshop in acupuncture that in many chronic conditions requiring extensive physiotherapy, the patient can be enabled to perform continuous simple and therapeutic exercises if the pain attendant upon the condition is alleviated through acupuncture anesthesia. Jerome Frank, however, in reporting upon his research in the placebo effect, opposed many forms of self-care, since his research indicates that a major variable in healing may be faith in the healer. Dr. Greenspan's presentation on applications of biofeedback indicated that much can be accomplished by providing the patient with specific and immediate information about his bodily state; he reported especially dramatic results wth stress-related disorders.

Dr. Levin and Mr. Milliken both talked about social dimensions of institutional health care with particular sensitivity to class and cultural issues. Milliken advocated understanding the nature of the institutions that deform social life for many Americans and destroy them as individuals, and Dr. Levin warned against normative health faddism in which the characteristics and needs of the majority of the client population could continue to be ignored. Both would agree that, in Dr. Levin's words, "We don't need to put more doctors in the South Bronx as much as we need to put more of the South Bronx into the doctors."

SOME EDITORIAL COMMENTS
ON THE IMPLICATIONS OF THE HOLISTIC HEALTH MOVEMENT

The Asian American Health and Mental Health Task Force is going to be addressing many of the issues that were raised at the meeting reported here. I feel that there are some serious implications for Asian minorities of the political momentum that can accrue to a unified health reform movement.

There is no way of separating ethical from scientific issues where health care for an underserved minority is concerned. But the rights and wrongs of the ethical situation are not all entirely clear, and bear some examination.

It is particularly important to recognize that American ethical judgments arise from a profoundly Western orientation. Thus, in reading between the lines of this report, a distinctly individualistic strain may be discerned. The human potential movement, with its focus on self-control, self-development, individual liberation from confining roles, and total responsibility for one's own actions, was much in evidence at the meeting. These values are all worthy and deserve serious attention, but when uncritically used to provide a charter for social policy, they can backfire in unfortunate ways. For example, totally ignored in this tradition is the inseparability of notions of the self from a much wider process of family and community involvement for many Asians and other members of non-Western traditions. This very popular and widely consumed form of psychologistic thinking is integral to the foundation of self-care as it has been evolving in the U.S., and as such has obviously made an important contribution to the health reform movement. (See the remarks of Dr. Levin above.) But it would be regrettable if a strongly normative individualistic ethic were to creep into the health care delivery systems as a whole; one can foresee it producing only guilt, confusion, and ineffective activity in many quarters.

A related concern of mine is the emphasis on "positive thinking" and "original innocence" peddled by many. As an aspect of the thoroughly valid idea that traditional distinctions between mental and physical realms of human activity must be abandoned, it seems natural to prescribe positive thinking as a cure for a variety of "holistic" ills. Nevertheless, it is very easy to apply such a concept in a vulgarly normative way, such that negative thoughts are held to be unnatural and not good for you, thus giving rise to further negative thoughts in the form of guilt. One also is led to wonder whether honesty and realistic thinking have become passe as standards of human behavior.

One of the earliest ideas to arise from the health reform movement was that medical care has been too illness-focused, and that what is needed is a definition of health. This must be one of the most problematic ideas in the history of medicine, and yet it must be dealt with, since it is obviously fundamental to the project of developing prevention-oriented health-care systems and dealing with life-style related illness. Two ideas that surfaced often at the meeting must be warned against, however; one is the search for "a definition of the optimal human being," a programme which if taken seriously would entail a completely unwarranted expansion of the health ethic into every aspect of social policy; it could uncritically mobilize the cultural and class values of the powerful to oppress non-"healthist" segments of the population under the unchallengeable banner of Health. Such extremes of thinking about health reform must be avoided. Reform should be for people, not of people.

For the same reason, the second extreme approach to defining "health" must be approached with caution, that being the concept of "high level wellness." This idea has arisen from the physical fitness movement, and seems to have led some health reformers to believe that almost everybody is chronically ill, no matter how symptom-free. Though the increased popular interest in sports and good nutrition, anti-smoking campaigns and weight loss programs, are no doubt making a positive contribution to the general health of Americans, we must resist too much life-style moralizing on the policy level. There is simply no way of knowing where sound medical advice ends and cultural imperialism begins, and "high level wellness" as a goal for the masses could easily mask much too large a dose of the latter.

The gist of these remarks on the holistic health movement and its relevance to Asian Americans is that health care professionals and reformers should be careful not to take themselves too seriously. In spite of the fact that all of us would like to save the world, it remains unclear just what a "saved" world would look like.

Many good ideas for responsible health system reform were proposed at the meeting, each of which can be carefully assessed from an Asian American perspective and, as such ideas are refined and implemented, evaluated from the same viewpoint and rejected if necessary. As Buckminster Fuller reminded the conference participants, good design (of social programs) is always the result of casting about for results through trial and error. Little can be gained by an uncritical and unswerving attachment to lofty principles in developing systems that are truly appropriate to the extremely diverse population that must be served.

It is also important to remember that "the enemy" in medical practice always wins in the end. As Dr. Levin remarked, "From one viewpoint, life is just a process of choosing a cause of death."

Bibliography

Adler, David A., Daniel J. Levinson and Boris M. Astrachan
1978   "The Concept of Prevention in Psychiatry." Archives of
        General Psychiatry 35:786-789 (June).

Amaranto, Ernesto A.
1978   "Mental Health Study of Filipino Immigrants in the New
        York Metropolitan Area." SIR Report No. 13. Chicago:
        Asian American Mental Health Research Center.

Arimoto, Mary M.
1975   "Formative Evaluation of Reaching Out. Service to Asian
        Women, July 1, 1973-June 1975." Long Beach, California:
        West Side Neighborhood Center.

Arkoff, Abe, Falak Thaver and Leonard Elkind
1966   "Mental Health and Counseling Ideas of Asian and Ameri-
        can Students." Journal of Counseling Psychology 13(2):
        219-223.

Belloc, Nedra B., Lester Breslow and Joseph R. Hochstim
1971   "Measurement of Physical Health in a General Population
        Survey." American Journal of Epidemiology 93(8):328-336.

Bennett, Charles G.
1973   "Mortality Trends in Hawaii, 1908-1962." R & S Report
        Issue No. 2:1-15 (April). Research and Statistics Office,
        Hawaii State Department of Health.

Berk, Bernard B. and Lucie Hirata
1973   "Mental Illness Among the Chinese: Myth or Reality?"
        Journal of Social Issues 29(2):149-166.

Berkman, Paul
1971   "Measurement of Mental Health in a General Population
        Survey." American Journal of Epidemiology 94(2):
        105-111.

Burch, Thomas
1975   "Trends in Cancer Mortality by Race in Hawaii 1910-
        1970." R & S Report Issue No. 7:1-20 (December). Re-
        search and Statistics Office, Hawaii State Department of
        Health.

1976   "Magnitude of Sudden Infant Death in Hawaii, 1968-
        1975." R & S Report Issue No. 10:1-7 (May). Research
        and Statistics Office, Hawaii State Department of Health.

1977   "Health of Residents, Immigrants and Inmigrants in
        Hawaii, 1973. A Report Based on The Hawaii Health
        Survey." R & S Report Issue No. 14:1-9 (April). Research
        and Statistics Office, Hawaii State Department of Health.

1977   "The Relationship Between Short Pregnancy Interval and
        Neonatal Death in Hawaii, 1968-1975." R & S Report
        Issue No. 15:1-10 (August). Research and Statistics Of-
        fice, Hawaii State Department of Health.

1977   "Chronic Illness and Hospitalization by Ethnicity and
        Income in the State of Hawaii: 1969-1971." R & S Report
        Issue No. 19:1-26 (December). Research and Statistics
        Office, Hawaii State Department of Health.

1978   "Ethnicity and Health in Hawaii, 1975". R & S Report
        Issue No. 23:1-6 (August). Research and Statistics Office,
        Hawaii State Department of Health.

Chan, Samuel Q.
    1976   "Services for the Developmentally Disabled: A Study of
            Asian Clients Within a Regional Center System." Uni-
            versity of California at Los Angeles. Mimeograph.

Chen, Alan
    1978   "Survey of the Usage of Health Care Facilities by the
            Chinese Residents in Chicago's Chinatown." Unpublished
            paper.

Chen, Martin K.
    1976   "Two Forms of an Equity Index for Health Resource Al-
            location to Minority Groups." Inquiry 13(3):228-232 (Sep-
            tember).

Chernow, Ron
    1973   "Chinatown, Their Chinatown: The Truth Behind the Fa-
            cade." New York 6(24):39-45 (June 11).

Conroy, John
    1978   "The Dark Side of Chinatown." Chicago 27(5):112 (May).

Cordova, Dorothy and Ick-Whan Lee
    1975   "Demonstration Project for Asian Americans: A Study of
            Problems of Asian Health Professionals." Seattle, Wash-
            ington: Demonstration Project for Asian Americans.

Dowling, Michael, Genie Kittlaus and Harold Confer
            "Major National Health Insurance Plans of the 94th Con-
            gress 1975." Copies may be obtained from Friends
            Committee on National Legislation, 245 2nd Street N.E.,
            Washington D.C. 20002.

Draguns, Juris, G., Linda Leaman and John M. Rosenfeld
    1971   "Symptom Expression in Christian and Buddhist Hospital-
            ized Psychiatric Patients of Japanese Descent in Ha-
            waii." Journal of Social Psychology 85:155-161.

Dunham, H. Warren
    1976   "Society, Culture and Mental Disorders." Archives of
            General Psychiatry 33:147-156 (February).

Elling, Ray, Russell Martin, Ronald Wintrob and Karen Greenwald
            "Health and Health Care in Hartford's North End. Re-
            port of the Health Action Survey." Unpublished paper.

Farquhar, Judith
    1977   "Why Do People Go or Don't Go to the Doctor." Bridge
            Magazine 5(3):48-51 (Fall).

Goldstein, Michael, Eliot H. Rodnick, Jerome R. Evans, Philip R. A.
    May and Mark R. Steinberg
    1978   "Drug and Family Therapy in the Aftercare of Acute
            Schizophrenics." Archives of General Psychiatry 35:1169-
            1177 (October).

Grupenhoff, John T.
    1978   1978 National Health Directory. Washington, D.C.:
            Science and Health Publications, Inc.

Haas, Michael
    1977   "Toward Equal Opportunity in Health Care. The Case of
            the Hawaii Department of Health, Mental Health Divi-
            sion." Photocopy.

Hackenberg, Robert A., Linda Gerber and Beverly H. Hackenberg
    1978   "Cardiovascular Disease Mortality Among Filipinos in
            Hawaii: Rates, Trends and Associated Factors." R & S
            Report Issue No. 24:7-14 (September). Research and
            Statistics Office, Hawaii State Department of Health.

Haug, James
    1976   "The Foreign Medical Graduate in American Surgery."
            Bulletin of the American College of Surgeons 61(4):7-9
            (April).

Health Care Institute
    1978   "A Proposal for Funding of a Primary Health Care Service
            Program as a Cost Control Demonstration Project." De-
            troit, Michigan.

Homma-True, Reiko
    1976   "Characteristics of Contrasting Chinatowns: 2. Oakland,
            California." Social Casework 57(3):155-159 (March).

Homma-True, Reiko, Trina Nahm, Serena Chen, Steve Ow-Ling,
Mark Mizuno, Wilma Louis and Irene Ortiz
    1975?   "Explorations of Mental Health Needs in an Asian Ameri-
            can Community: Review of Oakland's Asian Community
            Mental Health Services Client Data, June 30, 1975."
            Photocopy.

Ibrahim, I. B., C. Carter, D. McLaughlin and M. Rashad
    1977   "Ethnicity and Suicide in Hawaii." Social Biology 24(1):
            10-16 (Spring).

Iga, Mamoru
    1957   "The Japanese Social Structure and the Source of Mental
            Strains of Japanese Immigrants in the United States."
            Social Forces 35(3):271-278 (March).

Ikeda, Kiyoshi, Harry V. Ball and Douglas S. Yamamura
    1962   "Ethnocultural Factors in Schizophrenia--The Japanese in
            Hawaii." American Journal of Sociology 68(2):242-248
            (September).

Jenkins, Shirley and Barbara Morrison
    1978   "Ethnicity and Service Delivery." American Journal of
            Orthopsychiatry 48(1):160-165 (January).

JWK International Corporation
    1976   "Identification of Problems in Access to Health Services
            and Health Careers for Asian Americans." Vols. I, II and
            III. Submitted to the Office of Health Resources Oppor-
            tunity, Health Resources Administration, DHEW, July 31.

Katz, Martin M., Howard Godeman and Kenneth Sanborn
1969 "Characterizing Differences in Psychopathology Among Ethnic Groups: A Preliminary Report on Hawaii-Japanese and Mainland American Schizophrenics." Pp. 140-163 in William Caudill and Tsung-Yi Lin (eds.), Mental Health in Asia and the Pacific. Honolulu: University of Hawaii Press.

Kennedy, Edward
1977 "Health Security Act." Congressional Record, 95th Congress, January 11.

Kim, H. A.
1976 "Transplantation of Psychiatrists from Foreign Cultures." Journal of the American Academy of Psychoanalysis 4(1):105-112.

King, Haitung
1974 "Selected Epidemiologic Aspects of Major Diseases and Causes of Death Among Chinese in the United States and Asia." Pp. 487-550 (Chapter 31) in Arthur Kleinman et al. (eds.), Medicine in Chinese Cultures: Comparative Studies of Health Care in Chinese and Other Societies. DHEW Publication No (NIH)75-653. Bethesda, Maryland: John E. Fogarty International Center, National Institutes of Health.

King, Haitung and Frances B. Locke
1980 "A Century of Occupational Transition Among the Chinese in the United States." International Migration Review 14(1):15-42 (Spring).

King, Haitung and Haenszl Williams
1973 "Cancer Mortality Among Foreign- and Native-Born Chinese in the United States." Journal of Chronic Disease 26:623-646.

Kinzie, J. David
1974 "A Summary of Literature on Epidemiology of Mental Illness in Hawaii." Pp. 8-12 in Wen-Shing Tseng, John McDermott Jr., and Thomas Maretzki (eds.), Peoples and Cultures in Hawaii. Department of Psychiatry, University of Hawaii School of Medicine.

Koseki, Lawrence K.
1973 "Asian American Mental Health: An Asian American View." Paper presented at the American Psychiatric Association Meeting held in Honolulu, Hawaii, May 10.

Kuo, Wen
    1976   "Theories of Migration and Mental Health: An Empirical
            Testing on Chinese-Americans." Social Science and Medi-
            cine 10:297-306.

Kuwabara, Haruo and Reiko Homma-True
    1976   "National Social Policy Toward the Mentally Ill in Japan
            and its Consequences." International Journal of Mental
            Health 5(3):95-108 (Fall).

McCain, John
    1976   "A Multivariate Analysis of Statistics on the Hawaiian
            Community." R & S Report Issue No. 8:1-19 (January).
            Research and Statistics Office, Hawaii State Department
            of Health.

Maretzki, Thomas and Linda D. Nelson
    1969   "Psychopathology Among Hawaii's Japanese: A Compara-
            tive Study." Pp. 164-177 in William Caudill and Tsung-Yi
            Lin (eds.), Mental Health Research in Asia and the Pa-
            cific.   Honolulu: University of Hawaii Press.

Marsella, Anthony J., David Kinzie and Paul Gordon
    1973   "Ethnic Variations in the Expression of Depression."
            Journal of Cross-Cultural Psychology 4(4):435-458 (De-
            cember).

Marsella, Anthony J., Michael D. Murray and Charles Golden
    1974   "Ethnic Variations in the Phenomenology of Emotions: I.
            Shame." Journal of Cross-Cultural Psychology 5(3):312-
            328 (September).

Marsella, Anthony J., Kenneth O. Sanborn, Velma Kameoka, Lanette
Shizuri and Jerry Brennan
    1975   "Cross-Validation of Self-Report Measures of Depression
            Among Normal Populations of Japanese, Chinese and
            Caucasian Ancestry." Journal of Clinical Psychology
            31(2):281-287 (April).

Marsella, Anthony J., Lanette Shizuru, Velma Kameoka, Jerry Brennan and Kenneth O. Sanborn
    n.d.   "The Relationship Between Depression and Body-Image
            Satisfaction as a Function of Ethno-Cultural Group Mem-
            bership and Gender." University of Hawaii. Photocopy.

Marsella, Anthony J., Elaine Walker and Frank Johnson
    1973   "Personality Correlates of Depressive Disorders in Female
            College Students of Different Ethnic Groups." Inter-

national Journal of Social Psychiatry 19(1/2):77-81
(Spring/Summer).

Mass, Amy Iwasaki
1976 "Asians as Individuals: The Japanese Community." Social
Casework 56(3):160-164 (March).

The Nation's Health
1976 "Policy Statement Offered for the American Public
Health Association." September: 5-12.

Okano, Yukio
n.d.   "Japanese Americans and Mental Health. An Exploratory
Study of Attitudes." Photocopy.

Onoda, Lawrence
1977 "Neurotic-Stable Tendencies Among Japanese-American
Sanseis and Caucasian Students." Journal of Non-White
Concerns July: 180-185.

Owan, Tom
1975 "Asian Americans: A Case of Benighted Neglect." Occasional Paper No. 1. Chicago: Asian American Mental
Health Research Center.

Philpot, Terry
1978 "Asians and the NHS." Nursing Mirror 147(2):9 (July 13).

Ponce, Danilo E. and Vincent Lee
1977 "Intraethnic Violence in Hawaii School: A Mental Health
Consultation Experience." American Journal of Ortho-
psychiatry 47(3):451-455 (July).

Public Health Reports
1977 "Determining Ethnic Origin in an Interview Survey:
Problems and Recommendations." 92(5):414-420 (Sep-
tember-October).

Reed, Dwayne, Darwin Labarthe and Reuel Stallones
1970 "Health Effects of Westernization and Migration Among
Chamorros." American Journal of Epidemiology 92(2):
94-112.

Reed, T. E.
1976 "Alcohol and Acetaldehyde Metabolism in Caucasian,
Chinese and Americans." Canadian Medical Association
Journal 115:851-855 (November 6).

62   Bibliography

Regier, Darrel A., Irving D. Goldberg and Carl A. Taube
  1978   "The De Facto U.S. Mental Health Services System: A
         Public Health Perspective." Archives of General Psy-
         chiatry 35:685-693 (June).

Rhee, Sang-O, Thomas Lyons and Beverly Payne
  1978   "Patient Race and Physician Performances: Quality of
         Medical Care, Hospital Admissions and Hospital Stays."
         Draft copy.

Sata, Lindbergh S.
  1978   "A profile of Asian-American Psychiatrists." American
         Journal of Psychiatry 135:(4):448-451 (April).

Sato, Masayuki
  1979   "Shame: Paradoxical Affects and the Mental Health of
         Asian Americans." Paper presented at the California
         State Psychological Association Convention held in
         Monterey, California, February 8-11.

Shaw, Robert
  n.d.   "Health Services in a Disaster: Lessons from the 1975
         Vietnamese Evacuation." Photocopy.

  1977   "Preventive Medicine in the Vietnamese Refugee Camps
         on Guam." Military Medicine 141(1):19-28 (January).

Sheppard, Charles, Elizabeth Ricca, John Fracchia and Sidney Merlis
  1976   "Chemotherapeutic Choices of Native and Foreign Psy-
         chiatrists: Preference for an Acute Psychotic Episode."
         Psychological Reports 39:343-350.

  1976   "Chemotherapeutic Preference of Native and Foreign
         Specialists: A Move toward Consensus." Comprehensive
         Psychiatry 17(5):617-622.

Sheppard, James D.
  1976   "Minority Perspective of a National Health Insurance."
         Journal of National Medical Association 68(4):285-288
         (July).

Shibasaki, Hiroshi, Michael M. Okihiro and Yoshigoro Koroiwa
  1978   "Multiple Sclerosis Among Orientals and Caucasians in
         Hawaii: A Reappraisal." Neurology 28(2):113-118 (Feb-
         ruary).

Bibliography 63

Shu, Ramsay
1976 "Utilization of Mental Health Facilities: The Case for Asian Americans in California." Occasional Paper No. 4. Chicago: Asian American Mental Health Research Center.

Smith, Kline and French Laboratories
1977 Cultural Issues in Contemporary Psychiatry.

Sue, Derald Wing
1976 "Barriers to Effective Cross-Cultural Counseling." Paper presented at the Cross-Cultural Counseling Program held at the Culture Learning Institute, East-West Center, University of Hawaii, August 4-25.

1977 "Counseling the Culturally Different: A Conceptual Analysis." Personnel and Guidance Journal 55(7):422-425 (March).

Sue, Derald Wing and Austin C. Frank
1973 "A Typological Approach to the Psychological Study of Chinese and Japanese American College Males." Journal of Social Issues 29(2):129-148.

Sue, Derald Wing and David Sue
1976 "Ethnic Minorities: Failures and Responsibilities of Social Sciences." Paper presented at the Asian American Caucus Symposium of the California Personnel and Guidance Association held in Santa Barbara, California, September 10-12.

Sue, Stanley
1974 "Personality and Mental Health: A Clarification." Amerasia Journal 2(2):173-177 (Fall).

1975 "Delivery of Services to Dispersed Asian and Pacific Island Populations." Paper prepared for the National Project on Asian and Pacific Island Americans, U.S. Commission on Civil Rights, August.

1977 "Community Mental Health Services to Minority Groups-- Some Optimism, Some Pessimism." American Psychologist 32(8):616-624 (August).

1977 "Issues in the Training of Asian American Psychologists." Paper presented at the Annual Meeting of the American Psychological Association held in San Francisco, California, August.

1977   "Psychological Theory and Implications for Asian Americans." Personnel and Guidance Journal 55(7):381-389 (March).

Sue, Stanley and Derald Sue
1971   "Chinese American Personality and Mental Health." Amerasia Journal 1(2):36-49 (July).

Tan, Kong Meng
1973   "Foreign Trained Physicians in Illinois." Illinois Medical Journal 144(6):555-559 (December).

1977   "Foreign Medical Graduate Performance--A Review." Medical Care 15(10):882-829.

Thaver, Falak, Abe Arkoff and Leonard Elkind
1964   "Conceptions of Mental Health in Several Asian and American Groups." Journal of Social Psychology 62:21-27.

Tsushima, William T. and Jerome I. Boyer
1975   "Cross-Validation of the Halstead-Reitan Neuropsychological Battery: Application in Hawaii." Hawaii Medical Journal 34(3):94-96.

Tung, Tran Minh
1975   "The Vietnamese and Their Mental Health Problems: A Vantage View." Paper presented at the Meeting of the District of Columbia Chapter of the Washington Psychiatric Society and of the Medical Society of the District of Columbia held in Washington, D.C., October 1.

Udry, Richard J., Naomi M. Morris and Karl E. Bauman
1976   "Changes in Women's Preferences for the Racial Composition of Medical Facilities, 1969-74." American Journal of Public Health 66(3):284-286 (March).

U.S. Department of Health, Education and Welfare
1975   Proceedings of the International Conference on Women in Health, June 16-18, 1975. DHEW Publication (HRA) 76-51. Washington, D.C.: U.S. Government Printing Office.

1977   National Health Insurance National Outreach Report. Stock No. 817-961-10. Washington, D.C.: U.S. Government Printing Office.

U.S. Department of Health, Education and Welfare; Public Health Service
1978   Health, United States, 1978. DHEW Publication No. (PHS) 78-1232.

U.S. Department of Health, Education and Welfare; Public Health Service; ADAMHA; National Institutes of Health
1978   "Public Suggestions for DHEW Health Research Principles." Volume prepared for the National Conference on Health Research Principles, October 3-4.

U.S. Department of Health, Education and Welfare; Public Health Service; Health Resources Administration
1975   Minorities and Women in the Health Fields: Applicants, Students and Workers. DHEW Publication No. (HRA) 76-22.

1978   Minorities and Women in the Health Fields: Applicants, Students and Workers. DHEW Publication No. (HRA) 79-22.

1978   A Report to the President and Congress on the Status of Health Professions Personnel in the United States. DHEW Publication No. (HRA) 78-93.

U.S. Department of Health, Education and Welfare; Public Health Service; Health Resources Administration; National Center for Health Statistics
1978   "Health Characteristics of Minority Groups, U.S. 1976." Advancedata 27:1-7 (April 14).

U.S. Department of Health, Education and Welfare; Region V
1977   National Health Insurance Region V Report on Public Comments.

U.S. President's Commission on Mental Health
1978   "Report of the Special Populations Subpanel on the Mental Health of Asian/Pacific Americans." Pp. 773- 819 in Vol. III, Task Panel Reports Submitted to the President's Commission on Mental Health. Stock Number 040-000-00390. Washington D.C.: U.S. Government Printing Office.

Vaughn, Christine and Julian Leff
1976   "The Measurement of Expressed Emotion in the Families of Psychiatric Patients." British Journal of Social and Clinical Psychology 15:157-165.

Walters, William E.
1977   "Community Psychiatry in Tutuila, America Samoa."
        American Journal of Psychiatry 134(8):917-919.

Washington State Commission on Asian American Affairs
1977   "A Report on a Conference of Delegates from Indochinese
        Associations in Washington State." Seattle, Washington,
        September 24.

Weaver, Jerry
1978   "Public Policy Responses to the Health Needs of Asian
        American Families." Pp. B118-B158 in Summary and
        Recommendations, Conference on Pacific and Asian
        American Families and HEW-Related Issues. Stock No.
        017-000-00212-1. Washington, D.C.: U.S. Government
        Printing Office.

Wegner, Eldon L.
1977   "Chronic Illness and Hospitalization by Ethnicity and
        Income in the State of Hawaii: 1969-1971." R & S Report
        Issue No. 19:1-26 (December). Research and Statistics
        Office, Hawaii State Department of Health.

Weiner, Betsy Platt and Robert C. Marvit
1977   "Schizophrenia in Hawaii. Analysis of Cohort Risk in a
        Multi-Ethnic Population." British Journal of Psychiatry
        131:497-503.

White, Earnestine Huffman
1977   "Giving Health Care to Minority Patients." Nursing Clin-
        ics of North America 12(1):27-40 (March).

Williams, Kathleen N. and Robert H. Brook
1974   "Migration of Foreign Physicians to the United States: The
        Perspective of Health Manpower Planning." International
        Journal of Health Services 4(2):213-243.

1975   "Foreign Medical Graduates and Their Impact on the
        Quality of Medical Care in the United States." Santa
        Monica, CA: Rand Corporation.

Woods, Ernest and Herbert L. Gravitz
1976   "A Multiethnic Approach to Peer Counseling." Profes-
        sional Psychology May: 229-235.

Yamamoto, Joe, Quinton C. James and Normal Palley
1968   "Cultural Problems in Psychiatric Therapy." Archives of
        General Psychiatry 19:45-49 (July).

Yanagida, Evelyn and Anthony J. Marsella
  1977 "Discrepancy Among Different Generations of Japanese-American Women." Honolulu: University of Hawaii. Unpublished paper.

Yano, Katsuhiko, George G. Rhoads and Abraham Kagan
  1977 "Epidemiology of Serum Uric Acid Among 8,000 Japanese American Men in Hawaii." Journal of Chronic Diseases 30(3):171-184.

Yeh, Eng-Kung and Hung-Ming Chu
  1974 "The Image of Chinese and American Character: Cross-Cultural Adaptation by Chinese Students." Pp. 220-216 in William P. Lebra (ed.), Youth, Socialization, and Mental Health. Vol. III of Mental Health Research in Asia and the Pacific. Honolulu: University of Hawaii Press.